help yourself heal

yourself

heal

with

self-hypnosis

Linda Mackenzie

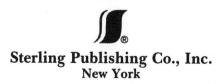

Sterling Publishing Co., Inc.
New York

Library of Congress Cataloging-in-Publication Data
Mackenzie, Linda.
  Help yourself heal with self-hypnosis / Linda Mackenzie.
    p. cm.
  Includes index.
  ISBN 0-8069-4969-4
    1. Autogenic training. 2. Self-care, Health. I. Title.
  RC499.A8 M336 2000
  615.8512—dc21
                                                        99-087964

10 9 8 7 6 5 4 3 2 1

Published by Sterling Publishing Company, Inc.
387 Park Avenue South, New York, N.Y. 10016
©2000 by Linda Mackenzie
Distributed in Canada by Sterling Publishing
c/o Canadian Manda Group, One Atlantic Avenue, Suite 105
Toronto, Ontario, Canada M6K 3E7
Distributed in Great Britain and Europe by Cassell PLC
Wellington House, 125 Strand, London WC2R 0BB, England
Distributed in Australia by Capricorn Link (Australia) Pty Ltd.
P.O. Box 6651, Baulkham Hills, Business Centre, NSW 2153, Australia

Sterling ISBN 0-8069-4969-4

Disclaimer: The following information is intended for general informa-tion purposes only. Individuals with health problems should always see their health care provider before administering any suggestions made in this book. Any application of the materials set forth in the following pages is at the reader's discretion and is his or her sole responsibility.

I would like to dedicate this book to Barbara E. Savin for her encouragement, advice, patience, and friendship. She reminds me to look at myself with laughter, whenever I get too serious. And to my daughter, Lisa Reitinger, who makes a difference in the world.

Most of all this book is dedicated to the seekers of self-empowerment and knowledge, for self-empowerment and knowledge reach out to destroy fear and negative thought — which are the only things that stand in the way of the accomplishment of one's desires.

ACKNOWLEDGMENTS

There are so many people who consciously and unconsciously contributed to this book that it is impossible to mention them all. However, I'd like to thank a few who have donated their time and knowledge to this endeavor: Barbara Savin, for her years of expertise in vitamins and supplements; Dr. Jung Min Kim, for sharing his knowledge of herbal medicine and acupuncture; Dr. Art Karno, for providing information on chiropractic care and homeopathy; Dr. Dan Condron, for his work on mental attitude and healing; and especially Steve Parker, MFCC, who introduced me to the world of healing hypnosis so many years ago.

Contents

CHAPTER 1

What Is Self-Hypnosis?

It has been proven that there is a mind-body connection. Self-hypnosis is a method that allows you to access this connection for the purpose of helping yourself. All hypnosis is an altered state of relaxed consciousness, between wakefulness and sleep, where ideas are accepted by suggestion rather than by logical evaluation. Self-hypnosis means you are placing yourself into this hypnotic state.

Many people associate hypnosis with stage shows and think that it is perhaps mystical or dangerous. In fact the opposite is true. Hypnosis is not a mind control method where a "victim" gives up his or her control. It actually helps you gain *more* control of your own life. Some people believe that you need to be gullible or weak-minded to be able to use hypnosis. This theory is also not true. People with above-average intelligence actually are better at using self-hypnosis techniques. Self-hypnosis is one of the most powerful tools that you can use to accomplish your goals. It helps you discover hidden skills and resources that you may not even be aware of.

SUGGESTION

Self-hypnosis uses the power of suggestion. Suggestion is a powerful motivator which we have been exposed to since childhood, which forms habitual behavior and attitudes. Our own personal belief system is based upon the accumulation of suggestions that we process throughout life. The ability to reason usually comes around the age of five. The conscious mind develops, and the child selects what is believed to be truth based on his or her emotions and experience. We learn to create our own perception of reality from patterns of repetition and their association with rewards and punishments. Reality is just our perception of what reality is. In essence, we become what we think. If we can take our perception of reality and change it with positive suggestion, we can then change that reality into one that is more conducive to overall health and well-being.

We accept suggestions that come in verbal and nonverbal forms.

When your mother told you: "Eat your spinach!" that was a direct command and a verbal suggestion. Body language is a form of indirect suggestion. For example, you smile, and someone smiles back at you. Suggestions can also be implied — for example, a nod of your head in concurrence to an idea or from someone you respect, such as a parent or teacher. Emotional suggestions can affect our emotional state by setting off emotions that are associated with an event. For example, someone you care about tells you he or she loves you, and you feel a sensation of happiness. Society can dictate suggestions that appeal to a person's desire to belong to a group — for example, when the fashion industry dictates the latest styles for people to wear. There are even environmental suggestions — a sunny day may make you feel happy.

Most important in the development of our perception of reality is whether negative or positive suggestion is used. Since we are what we think, it is important to use positive suggestions and not negative ones. Negative suggestions limit the scope of your reality, inhibit change, and create contradictory patterns that can stop you from achieving what you want. Positive suggestions allow you to be open to accept change and renewal. They allow opportunity to knock on your door to provide you with a plethora of options for making your reality into one that flows with life and can include physical, emotional, and spiritual healing. In the matter of self-healing, positive suggestions are delivered through the self-hypnosis method to access the mind-body connection, which helps effect change in your body to boost it back to health.

HYPNOTIC TRANCE

What does it feel like being in a hypnotic, trancelike state? A good example is: You are driving along daydreaming and are not aware of the usual things that are happening around you; suddenly you come to a stoplight, which jars you back to reality. The way you feel when daydreaming is how you feel when in a hypnotic trance. Another example: You are watching a television program and are so engrossed that you forget about the time; suddenly the program is over. In both situations you are in control and aware of the things around you, but your mind has been concentrating on something else. The main difference between these trancelike experiences and a self-hypnotic trance is that in a self-hypnotic trance, you consciously use positive suggestions to motivate you towards a specific goal. In hypnotic trance, you are not in a sleep state, but merely in a different state, which allows a direct flow of suggestions to enter into your subconscious mind without criticism.

SELF-HYPNOSIS

All hypnosis is self-hypnosis, and almost everyone can use and do self-hypnosis. Since everyone is different, each person will experience hypnosis in his or her own particular way. I believe that the only limits to self-hypnosis are the limits you place upon yourself. You can help yourself heal and decrease or eliminate symptoms of illness and emotional disease with self-hypnosis.

Take my own case history with chronic fatigue syndrome. In 1987, I was attacked by the virus. I developed symptoms of panic attacks, spoke in distorted sentences, had low grade fevers, ear imbalance, vision changes, flulike symptoms, and I needed to sleep 16 to 18 hours a day. The medical doctors were baffled. I was shuffled off from one specialist to the next for five months, until they came up with the diagnosis. After the diagnosis, they said there was nothing they could do.

I decided at that point to take control and try self-healing. I changed my diet and started taking vitamins, supplements, and herbs. Then I went to a local hypnotherapist to see if hypnosis could help me heal. I was very surprised at the outcome. Within six weeks I was feeling much better; as I was now armed with self-hypnosis techniques, my physical symptoms started to disappear. After a period of time I was completely well. I was sold on self-hypnosis and I still am! I use it every time I start to feel ill or slip into a negative mode. The illness or negative emotion simply just disappears and is replaced by a feeling of such empowerment that it renews my sense of well-being. Self-hypnosis is a very powerful method to effect positive change.

There are many documented cases such as mine, where self-hypnosis has been proven to work against physical illness and emotional problems. Since self-hypnosis can play such an important role in healing, let's take a look at how it works.

MIND-BODY CONNECTION

We hear a lot about the mind-body connection, but what really is this connection? How can we use self-hypnosis to access this connection to help reach our goals of health and well-being? When we have an emotion, it produces a feeling, which turns into a physical sensation. For example: You are watching a horror movie and you start to feel afraid, so goosebumps appear on your skin. In this case you got an emotion (fear) that turned into a feeling (being afraid) and became a physical sensation (goosebumps). We all have this mind-body connection. Self-hypnosis uses positive suggestions or images to produce positive emotions to produce positive sensations in the body to aid in self-healing.

Let's try an exercise to see if this works for you. Get very relaxed and centered. Start breathing slowly. Imagine there is a large glass of 100% pure lemon juice in front of you. Imagine yourself picking up the glass. Close your eyes for a moment and picture this glass. See the color, the shape, the liquid in the glass. Open your eyes. Now close your eyes again and imagine you're taking a great big sip from this glass of 100% pure lemon juice. Open your eyes. Did you get a sour taste in your mouth? Did your mouth water? Did you shudder?

This is one way self-hypnosis uses images to produce a physical sensation. You really didn't take a sip from that glass, yet your imagination allowed you to process the information it received, which gave you some sort of reaction.

SENSORY PERCEPTION

Each of us processes the world differently. Each person's unique subconscious mind, which has evolved since childhood, is the result of the special way each of us perceives the world with our three major senses: sight (visual), hearing (auditory), and touch (kinesthetic). Some people relate better to visual stimulation, while others relate more to auditory or kinesthetic stimulation. Although in reality we use all five senses at different times, including taste and smell, in learning, most of us gravitate towards using one of the three major senses predominantly. The person who is mainly visual can be heard to use phrases like, "I see," or "I really don't see it that way." Auditory people may say, "That doesn't sound too good," or "Listen to what happened." People who are mainly kinesthetic learn by feeling and may say things like, "I feel good today," or "I don't feel the same way as you." In imagery development, it is best to use a combination of all three of these senses — visual, auditory, and kinesthetic — to maximize your success.

POSITIVE IMAGERY

Positive imagery is an important part of suggestion in self-hypnosis. The more you are involved in the process, the better it will work for you. Use the self-hypnosis scripts in this book, but don't limit yourself to them. Incorporate your own personal positive experiences, so that your unconscious mind can work quickly and specifically on your problem. In dealing with self-healing, you will be more successful if you know the what, where, why and how of your body's problem. Then, by using visualization, you can target these specific areas of your problem and get your body's internal defense systems to work with you at maximum efficiency. This will speed your healing process, so learn how your illness or emotional disease affects your physical body and always use positive imagery without self-criticism or self-doubt.

Self-hypnosis can aid self-healing, but you must work on a mind-body-spirit level to fully conquer your problem. All are equally important. When you are ill, positive thinking and positive emotions are necessary for the mind to work at its fullest potential. Eating right; taking the right supplements, herbs, vitamins, and minerals; getting enough rest; and doing what's right for your body are all significant in aiding the body's part in the healing process. The spirit, or maintaining the desire to heal, becomes very significant to the whole process of self-healing. Magnificent results can be obtained, but it needs the cooperation of you as a total being with a total commitment on all levels to accomplish your desired results. Do not doubt that you can work miracles, because you can!

THE BRAIN

Let's take a look at how the brain works. The brain is divided into two parts: the left, logical side and the right, creative side. The left side deals with logic, words, and rational thought. The right side is the seat of our imagination and intuition. It is our creative side. Because of day-to-day circumstances, we usually are in a left, logical brain mode; however, to always be in a left-brain mode causes an imbalance in the brain. By yielding to the right, creative side of the brain, we can actually restore the brain's balance to access the mind-body connection to achieve what we want. Remember that your brain is a highly efficient system that is connected to every cell in your body by billions of connections. The way it processes information is twofold.

The first is that it takes notice of what's happening in the body and establishes what it should do to solve the problem. The second is that it takes action through both the right and left sides of the brain by sending out chemical, electrical, and mechanical messages to the other parts of the body.

The left, conscious mind is aware of and in contact with reality. It retrieves or gathers, sorts and tests information, makes a decision, and subsequently directs action. It then stores this information in the right, subconscious mind. Your conscious mind shuts down while you sleep, but it maintains control of your senses. Your right, subconscious mind controls the health and function of every system in your body. It is your problem solver. It actually automatically steers you towards your goal. It totally accepts the idea of what you want to accomplish without giving an opinion, and then acts upon on it without judgment. This is exactly why self-hypnosis targets the right, creative side, because it can do what we want.

It is a fact that we only use 10% of our brains. My independent theory is that if we learn to use and balance both sides of the brain more effectively, we create an access or pathway to the 90% of the subconscious brain that we don't consciously use. I believe that this part of the brain has the ability to promote self-healing, as well as increasing our higher intuitive abilities. Self-hypnosis is a tool you can use to balance the brain and tap into your inner ability to accomplish self-healing.

CHAPTER 2

Stress, Change, and Positive Thought

To effectively use self-hypnosis, we need to look at stress and how we cope with fear and change. If we learn about stress and the dynamics of change, we can maximize self-hypnosis methods to better facilitate a long-term healthier and happier life. In essence, we can minimize or eliminate some of the problems, keep them from recurring, and even stop them before they begin. Stress is the major culprit in illness and emotional disease.

STRESS

Stress is a more important factor today than it has ever been before. Some stress is good, because it helps us grow and keeps us motivated. In fact, every action or reaction we have comes from stress. However, too much stress causes emotional breakdowns, illness, and even premature death. In fact, 60% of all physicians' case loads are stress-related. The early warning signs of too much stress are expressed physically when your body experiences pain, your energy level changes, and you feel body sensations that vary from your normal sensations. Stress can be felt emotionally when you have too many negative emotions like anger, fear, sadness, or depression. Your normal mental processing may change, which can reveal itself by either an overactive or inactive mind. Your behavioral patterns can be expressed by overdoing or underdoing things, developing clutter, avoiding situations, or being too aggressive. These are some of the warning signs that there is too much stress in your life and that you need to eliminate it so that you don't become ill. The human reaction to stress has not changed since the days of the cave dweller. When a caveman was attacked by a large animal, he reacted in a fight or flight mode. He would either stand up and fight the animal or run away. We still use this same reaction today.

Four types of stress affect how we look, think, and feel. Everything that happens to us is caused by one or a combination of these stresses. When trying to identify the cause of illness or emotional disease, we must look at which stress or stresses are causing the problem. The four types of stress are:

1. Physical stress, which manifests itself in illness, lack of sleep, and bacterial, viral, or fungal infections.

2. Nutritional stress, which happens when your body isn't getting or digesting the right foods, supplements, vitamins and nutrients.

3. Emotional stress occurs when you have negative emotions such as grief, guilt, anger, or frustration.

4. Environmental stress is present when pollutants inside or outside your body affect your body or mind. Examples are alcohol, air pollutants, and prescription drugs that can cause physical and mental side effects.

To determine which stress or stresses are causing your problem, you have to associate your problem with one or more of the four types of stress. For example, you have an upset stomach. Is it because:

*Someone punched you in the stomach (physical stress)?

*Your body doesn't have enough enzymes to process food (nutritional stress)?

*Your boss just told you that your job is in jeopardy (emotional stress)?

*You got food poisoning (environmental stress)?

Effective stress diagnosis can help you decide which self-hypnosis scripts you should use to help you to have a better chance to conquer your problem.

Stress can be associated with the fear of change. Let's look at the movement, sources, and control of change to see how this affects our health.

CHANGE

Change is constant. Nothing stays the same, but it's interesting to note that change moves in an upward, cyclical movement. It's like a spiral going towards the sky. The only thing we can depend on is that things are going to change. You will never experience the same change in exactly the same way as before. There will always be something that is different, because we are constantly moving up that spiral as we learn more about life's lessons and ourselves. If change is constant, that means we are always in some form of change. Using self-hypnosis to manage the change in our lives can be very useful, especially in the case of illness and emotional disease. Change can be self-initiated, forced, anticipated, unexpected, or caused by making a decision or taking action. No matter where it comes from, we are always in one of the four stages of change.

Let's take a look at the four stages of change in association with illness and emotional disease. They are:

1. A flourishing time, when we feel totally healthy on a mind-body-spirit level.

2. A shifting time, when we know things are changing and something's not right.

3. An adaptation time or information-gathering time, when things are not happening as they usually are.

4. An action time, when we actually start doing something about getting well.

These cyclical stages repeat themselves over and over again on all levels, all the time. The trick is to use self-hypnosis at the shifting time to minimize the impact of the adaptation time so you can maximize the action time to get back to your flourishing time. However, no matter what stage you are in, self-hypnosis can make it easier to make the transition and help you through the stages of change faster. In fact, self-hypnosis is a very effective way to help you control and process change more effectively.

When learning to control change, timing factors come into play. Some changes can get instantaneous results, while others take some time. Although some people report results after the very first time they use self-hypnosis, it usually takes approximately six weeks to work. Don't get discouraged; self-hypnosis does work, but your body has its own internal clock that you have to train to work with your mind and your spirit. The more you practice, the better it will work.

Now that we have learned about the sources, stages, and control of change, we come to the most important part: How do we handle change? Do you view change as an ally or an enemy? Do you fear it, or welcome it as a new opportunity? You can look at it either way, but which way do you think brings less stress? Here is an insight for you: *Change is always positive.*

When you welcome change and make it your ally, you experience less stress on all levels, spend less time in crisis, and can use the extra energy you will free up to enhance your life. Even when we are going through difficult times or think a change is a negative experience, in retrospect we see that change always produces a positive experience. You always learn something about yourself. You always grow. Remember: we are what we think! So think positive.

POSITIVE THOUGHT

Even illness is a positive experience. In retrospect, my illness was the most positive experience of my life. I learned to balance my life in a more positive way. Before my illness, two things were "important" in my life: my career and my family. After the illness, I added spirituality and made it an active part of my life. I also included time for my friends, the community, and myself. My life became more balanced and fulfilling. I learned to live in the moment. Because of the plethora of symptoms, I did not have control of my body, so I gave up control, ego, expectations, and negative thinking. I learned to self-heal. This promoted me to a place I had never been in my life. For the first time I felt whole in body, mind, and spirit. Now I get to help people every day, which brings me tremendous joy. Even though going through my illness seemed negative at the time, the end result was positive.

KEEPING POSITIVE

It has been proven that negative emotions lower our immune system and keep us bogged down mentally. Having negative emotions delays and stops us from reaching our goals. They actually inhibit the brain in accomplishing what we want. Positive emotions actually boost the immune system and make the brain work in a more balanced mode, which is conducive to change. How do we keep positive and balance the brain? We can't keep positive if we try to control situations. This uses the left brain and puts the right brain out of balance. Trying to control situations actually creates a paradox or contradiction in the brain. Have you ever wanted something so much that it just didn't happen? That's because trying to control the situation makes your goals rigid and actually inhibits the mind-body connection from working to accomplish what you want. You also can't keep positive if you worry about what people think.

Remember that every person is coming from his or her own perception of reality. So whose reality is right? We need to recognize who we are and accept ourselves. Every one of us is special, and each person has special gifts. It is our choice whether we use them or not.

Don't confuse happiness with fulfillment of desires; this also inhibits positive thought. Wanting is natural in life, but the idea that we can't be happy unless we satisfy a certain desire is not!

Another trap against keeping positive is what I call "My way is the only right way!" or perpetual insistence that you are right all of the time. This insistence shows a small view of the world. It makes you feel safe, but stops communication and the ability to make a choice. "My way is the only right way" usually relies on anger and blame. These two negative emotions are used to create a perception of your independence. In truth all it does is cut you off from positive thought.

Rationalization is another way of thinking that helps eliminate positive thought. Rationalization means you assemble an explanation to conform to your perspective, but it has no foundation because you falsely attribute to others your own way of thinking, feeling, and acting. Remember, no two people are alike, so this strategy fails. When your head and your heart can't come together, it's called rationalization.

You can't keep positive if you use the words "I should." This is usually based on false social beliefs, which keep us plunged into negative feelings, not positive ones.

One of the biggest pitfalls to keeping positive is if we live in the past or the future. This helps to keep our minds fragmented and creates that contradiction or paradox in the brain. Remember that this stops us from accomplishing what we want to accomplish. You really can't do anything about the past, because it's over. The future has so many variables, so you really can't do anything about it either. By focusing on the past or the future, we focus on discontinuity. We establish fixed points to which we attach significance, projections, feelings, expectations, and attitudes. These become our goals, and we become rigid. When we are ill, our bodies need to work in a "go with the flow" mode. When we fix our thoughts on the past or the future, we are inhibiting our minds from focusing on healing our bodies. This gets in the way of the healing process, so the best place to be is here, right now, in this moment.

By living in the now and focusing on this moment, life flows in a natural pattern. We experience life more fully. We set up our goals of what we want to accomplish and then put our intention to work. Then just let it go so that it can be accomplished.

INTENTION

Intention is an important element of self-hypnosis. It tells your right, subconscious side of the brain what you want to accomplish. So what exactly is intention, and how can you get it to work for you?

We already know that trying to control situations (e.g., "I will get better!") won't work. Negative thinking ("I'll never get better," or "There's nothing I can do") won't work. Neither will worrying about what others think, trying to fulfill your desires, insisting that your way is the only way, using the words "I should," or rationalizing. Intention is not using the ego to set up significance, projections, feelings, expectations, and attitudes (e.g., "Tomorrow I know I'll feel 100% better because I'll get more sleep tonight").

All the normal, logical ways that our left, logical, conscious mind uses to solve problems have no effect on the right, creative subconscious. So what is intention? Intention is to: FEEL, KNOW AND TRUST THAT WHAT YOU WANT IS BEING ACCOMPLISHED! It really is that simple. Remember: your mind, body, and spirit are working 24 hours a day, 365 days a year to keep you healthy and happy. That's their job. By feeling, knowing, and trusting that your body will do its job and using self-hypnosis, your goals will be accomplished.

CHAPTER 3

How to Prepare for Self-Hypnosis

Successful self-hypnosis requires a combination of four equally important elements. These are: specific intention, responsibility, mental relaxation, and the self-hypnosis process. Once you have learned to put these elements to work, you will be in possession of one of the most powerful tools of your life: self-hypnosis.

SPECIFIC INTENTION

Self-hypnosis puts your intention to work. The success of your self-hypnosis will depend on how specific your intention is. What is your goal? Make sure you are clear about what it is. Also make sure it is achievable. If you are overweight by 400 lbs, you can't expect to lose 250 lbs overnight. Learn to set up clear, achievable, specific intentions; for example, "I want to lose 3 lbs in a week." Some of your goals may have to be reached in steps. You can accomplish them, but it will take some time. Remember that your subconscious mind is goal-driven and will react to your specific intention to bring about success.

The most effective intention usually is combined with a strong emotion. Let's take the example of having a headache. Ask yourself what is it that you want to change. "I want to stop headache pain." First, you need to really *feel* that you want your headache to go away. Second, you have to *know* that your right, creative, subconscious mind will work on this task. Third, you have to *trust* that the headache will go away. Whatever you believe is what your body will do.

A specific intention is:

* Clear   * Achievable

* You feel it   * You know it is happening

* You trust it is being accomplished.

RESPONSIBILITY

Using self-hypnosis without taking responsibility will prove to be futile and a waste of time. Knowing what you want to do and doing it are two different things. For self-hypnosis to work you must do it. Procrastination won't get you where you want to go. Placing responsibility on outside events or other people doesn't cut it either. We give away our personal power by not taking responsibility for our own actions. You and you alone are responsible for the conditions in your mind, body, and spirit. For example, doctors and health practitioners are there to help and guide you, but they are not responsible for your health — you are! You have to be willing to take this responsibility. If you are going to expend your energy on practicing self-hypnosis, then be persistent. Make a commitment towards what you want to accomplish, keep positive, and take the responsibility of doing it.

Although some people can see and feel the results of self-hypnosis after the very first time, it usually takes about six weeks. People are unique, and so is the way they process information. Don't get discouraged: self-hypnosis will work. Self-hypnosis can be practiced anytime, but I suggest doing it at least once in the morning and in the evening right before you go to bed.

Responsibility is:

* Being accountable to and for yourself
* Maintaining your personal power
* Making a commitment
* Being persistent
* Doing self-hypnosis regularly
* Keeping positive.

MENTAL RELAXATION

Mental relaxation is another major key to successful self-hypnosis. Relaxation is the body's and mind's "rest and restoration" period. A relaxed mental state provides you with direct access to your subconscious mind. When we are fully relaxed, our mental judgment and censors are turned off; that is the best time for our thoughts to get through to the subconscious. A relaxed state that is conducive to self-hypnosis is one that is without any tension. It is used before, during, and after the self-hypnosis process.

True relaxation is an art. Just as an artist prepares to paint a picture, so you must prepare to relax. Find a comfortable place, a place where it is quiet and you won't be disturbed. It may be a chair, a bed, or even the floor. Make sure that you are comfortable, your clothing is loose, your arms and legs are uncrossed, and you are in a comfortable position. Now become calm and focused. Empty your mind of all thoughts, and start to concentrate on the breath and breathing. Just focus on the breath and breathe deeply in through the nose and exhale from the mouth.

This activates the vagus nerve, which is the major quieting nerve in the body. This nerve runs from the medulla in the brain down to the base of the spine. It branches out to the heart, respiratory, and intestinal tracts. When we concentrate on the breath and breathe deeply, the vagus nerve goes into action. It immediately lowers our blood pressure, heart rate, respiratory rate, and pulse rate. Our natural response when we are angry or in many other stressful situations is to breathe deeply. This simply activates the vagus nerve to quiet the body.

If your body is resisting relaxation, start by tightening the muscles in each part of your body one by one. Hold each muscle as tight and tense as you can for five seconds and then release. Do this to each muscle in your body; don't forget that your head has muscles too! Then try centering again and focusing on the breath and breathing.

Now that your body is relaxed, we need to relax the mind. This is placing our minds into a deeper relaxation. Empty your mind of all thoughts. Don't get distracted. If a thought comes in, gently acknowledge it and let it pass by. Do not make judgments, just push it gently away. Do this as many times as you need to. Just relax and concentrate on the breath and breathing. If you use a script in this book, it will take you through this process.

Total relaxation steps:

* Find a quiet place

* Get comfortable

* Loosen clothing

* Uncross arms and legs

* Get centered

* Concentrate on the breath and breathing

* Totally relax your body

* Totally relax your mind.

SELF-HYPNOSIS PROCESS

The process of self-hypnosis includes finding a quiet, comfortable place, formulating your intention, getting centered, concentrating on the breath and breathing, relaxing the body, deepening relaxation to include the mind, implementing suggestions, and awakening.

We have covered most of the process in our previous chapters. Let's take a look at the awakening part of the process. If you use the scripts provided in this book, they will take you through this step.

AWAKENING

After completing the implementation of your suggestions, you may be ready to awaken. You can awaken at will; there is no danger of your not being able to awaken. You will feel relaxed, without body tension, and be very clear-minded. Just open your eyes when you are ready. Take a moment, relax, and enjoy yourself waking up from this restful state.

The self-hypnosis process is:

* Find a comfortable, quiet place

* Formulate your intention

* Get centered

* Concentrate on the breath and breathing

* Relax the body

* Deepen relaxation to include the mind

* Implement suggestion

* Awaken

* Feel, know, and trust that your intention is being accomplished.

There are from 1 to 4 self-hypnosis scripts given for each illness and emotional disease discussed in this book. Each of the scripts goes through the complete process. Everything you need is provided in these scripts. If you want to change my scripts to add something that is pertinent to you, this will not make them any less effective. You might want to try developing and using your own scripts; this can work too! The real key to self-hypnosis is to do it and to feel, know, and trust that it is working. I have included charts that may help boost your body back to health with suggestions on food and diet, vitamins and supplements, herbs, aromatherapy and the mental attitude that contributed to causing the problem.

Note: Herbs are potent natural medicines that need to be treated with knowledge and respect. Since each person's body processes substances differently, precautions must be taken when using herbs. If you are considering using herbs, thorough research is required as to what types and dosages are exactly right for you. Remember that drug interactions may occur if you are using other herbs or medications. Certain physical conditions, such as pregnancy, may warrant not using a particular herb. It is always wise to check with your health practitioner before starting any program, including an herbal one. Good luck and good health!

CHAPTER 4

Aging

Your body's physiological age can be much younger than your actual chronological age. Documented studies show that the potential of the human life span is 120 years. Aging involves biological, nutritional, emotional, and awareness factors that can affect a person's health and overall well-being.

The primary cause of biological aging is the loss of cells' ability to reproduce in quick succession. Our genetic makeup controls the life span of our cells and cellular reproduction. In fact, our genetic makeup is connected to all of the systems and functions of the body. Intricate chemical interactions in the body are responsible for production and maintenance of our hormones and immune system. As aging occurs, cell reproduction, hormones, and the immune system slow down. To reduce the aging process, the primary goals are to protect, repair, and maintain the body, including its cells and genetic makeup. This enhances the production of natural hormones. Diet, vitamins, minerals, and supplements can counteract biological aging by boosting the immune system, which helps the body to maintain itself and work at peak efficiency.

The secondary goals are to promote muscle strength, bone density, skin tightness, skin moistness, mental clarity, sexual function, positive moods, and to increase energy levels. This can be accomplished by exercise, proper diet, and stress elimination.

There are nutritional factors that contribute to aging. Nutrients are the building blocks of the body, which provide for its energy and repair. Digestive enzymes break down foods into nutrients. After the age of 40, digestive enzyme production decreases, which may result in improper digestion and poor absorption of nutrients. Poor dietary habits contribute to aging, because they create a lack of proper nutrients that are necessary for the body's maintenance. This lowers the immune system and affects mood. Proper diet and digestive enzyme supplements can help food digestion and absorption so the body can get proper nutrients and utilize them correctly to help combat aging.

Negative emotional factors contribute to aging by creating stress in the mind and body. Emotions such as worry, anger, regret, depression, lone-liness, grief, and self-criticism are negative. These negative emotions man-ifest or contribute to illness and disease in the body and lack of well-being. Numerous studies have shown that negative emotions lower our immune system and cause acceleration of aging, whereas positive emo-tions actually boost the immune system and combat aging. Approaching life with positive thought creates positive energy that flows through the body. It is this energy that enhances physical and emotional well-being. Remember: you are what you think.

The most positive tool against aging is awareness. One is not alone, but part of the intricate existence of life. Some of the general principles of awareness include: living in the moment, listening to intuition, helping others, taking responsibility to be the best you can be, maintaining con-sciousness of what's happening to and around you, inviting spirituality into your life, and eliminating fear, judgment, and expectations. Practicing these principles creates a happier life.

Taking care of the biological, nutritional, emotional, and awareness fac-tors will enhance the anti-aging process, improve health, and make you look, feel, and be younger.

Aging Relief Remedies

MENTAL ATTITUDE
Cause: refusal to envision newness of life.
Cure: try new things.

FOODS & DIET
Avoid: sugar, caffeine, nicotine, alcohol, artificial flavorings, colors, and preservatives.
Good Foods: grapefruit, spinach, tomatoes, strawberries, blueberries, yogurt, kelp, broccoli, cabbage, apricots, grapes, lamb, chicken, oats, molasses, corn, rye, yams, carrots, turnips, soybeans, sea algae, flaxseed oil, alfalfa, pumpkin seeds, and nuts.

VITAMINS & SUPPLEMENTS
Multivitamin and mineral supplement with whole foods and enzymes, Vitamin C, A, E, D, B complex, pantothenic acid, choline, amino acids, bioflavonoids, glutathione, L-lysine, L-tyrosine, L-arginine, melatonin, coenzyme Q10, SOD (superoxide desmutase), HGH (human growth hormone), DHEA (dehydroepiandrosterone), zinc, selenium, and grape seed extract.

HERBS
Wild yam, horsetail, burdock root, calendula, cumin, dill, parsley, garlic, licorice root, nettle, ginkgo biloba, green tea, ginseng, gotu kola, hawthorn berries, milk thistle.

AROMATHERAPY
Rose, lavender, chamomile.

Self-hypnosis is a very positive way to help you combat aging. The following scripts should be used in the morning and at night. To optimize results, you may even want to try the scripts for energy, general illness, memory, and stress.

AGE MANAGEMENT SCRIPTS

THE VIEW
Intention: To reduce the aging process.

Find a comfortable place where you won't be disturbed, and sit in a comfortable chair. Now sit back and relax with both feet on the floor, and place your hands on the armrests of the chair or in your lap — whichever is comfortable for you.

Concentrate as you breathe deeply, letting the air come into your nose and out your mouth. Concentrate and breathe IN with the nose and OUT with the mouth. IN with the nose and OUT with the mouth. And IN with the nose and OUT with the mouth. Now let's concentrate on breathing OUT with the mouth and IN with the nose. And OUT with the mouth and IN with the nose. And OUT with the mouth and IN with the mouth.

Imagine you are in the mountains. The sky is blue and the sun is shining brightly. Hear the birds in the trees around you. Smell the pungent, woodsy aroma of the plants. Everything around you is calm and peaceful. You are walking on a mountain trail. As you turn the corner, you see a very large flat rock. The rock is overlooking the most beautiful view you have ever seen. You are not in a rush and seem to be at one with your surroundings. So peaceful and calm. Sit down on the rock and look at the view. See how beautiful it is.

(Close your eyes for a moment and see the view.)

Feeling peaceful, you seem to drift away, becoming part of all you see. It is as if you are inside and outside of yourself at the same time. Feel the happiness and the freedom. In this special place you feel your body working correctly. You feel the shift as your body's aging clock seems to slow down. All the stress in the body is fading away as you sit so calmly, so relaxed in this time and place. You feel your body repairing itself. Every cell in the body reproducing and maintaining itself.

(Close your eyes for a moment and feel the repair of your body.)

Now you feel your hormones increasing to levels that are exactly right for you. Everything in your body is communicating correctly. The hypothalamus and pituitary glands adjusting and working so properly. You feel your skin tightening and being filled with the moisture it needs. Your bones, muscles and organs working properly and at full potential. How good you feel.

(Close your eyes for a moment and feel the changes taking place.)

Your digestive enzymes are now being balanced, and you feel how the nutrients are entering your body, giving your body the energy it needs. Feel how your immune system is working. It is at its top capacity, fighting off disease and illness. You feel and know that you are so healthy and everything is working as it should.

Your mood is filled with happiness and you feel the warmth of joy entering your body. The positive energy is flowing through your body. You are feeling good. Looking good. Feel your memory shifting as it becomes sharp and clear. You can think fast and with such clarity. How wonderful this is. The positive energy continues to move throughout your body, your mind. All your systems are working properly. The mind and body in perfect synchronicity.

Now start to center yourself, keeping the feeling of your perfectly working mind and body with you. Take a look at the view one last time. Get up off the rock and continue walking up the mountain trail. The sun is bright and warm. The air temperature is exactly right for you. As you turn around a bend in the trail, you see a babbling brook with a rock in the middle. In the brook tiny fishes swim silently and peacefully. Look at the rock. In the middle of the rock you see a clock. This is a magic clock that can turn back time. The hands of the clock can be moved. Turn the clock's hands backward. You know that as you do this you are setting your own biological clock back.

Turn back the hands of the clock until you feel that it is the right time for you. As you turn the hands backward, feel your body responding.

Your own internal clock deep within you is turning backwards. All the genes, the chromosomes, the DNA responding. Shifting. Adjusting.

(Close your eyes for a moment and feel this shift.)

When you are done, look down at the brook. Watch as the brook turns into a pond of clear still water. Look down into the water and see your image. Your skin is tighter, your eyes are bright, and all your stress is gone. You look younger and your body feels younger. Everything in perfect working order. Look at how young you are. How beautiful you are. You smile and feel so happy knowing that you have accomplished much today. This feeling will stay with you.

THE MAGICAL PLACE
Intention: To reduce aging and increase positive thought.

Find a comfortable place where you won't be disturbed, and sit in a comfortable chair. Now sit back and relax with both feet on the floor, and place your hands on the armrests of the chair or in your lap — whichever is comfortable for you.

Concentrate as you breathe deeply, letting the air come into your nose and out your mouth. Concentrate and breathe IN with the nose and OUT with the mouth. IN with the nose and OUT with the mouth. And IN with the nose and OUT with the mouth. Now let's concentrate on breathing OUT with the mouth and IN with the nose. And OUT with the mouth and IN with the nose. And OUT with the mouth and IN with the mouth.

Imagine you are asleep in a bed all by yourself. The bed is soft and comfortable and you feel so very safe. You are dreaming. In your dream is a magical place. As you look around this magical place you feel a sense of wonder and awe. Beautiful lights surround you and you feel so centered. Love seems to flow from inside and outside of you. It is all around and the feeling is so incredible. You know you are not alone but part of this wonderful love. Part of the plan for this wonderful life.

(Close your eyes for a moment and feel this love.)

Start walking in this magical land. You see in front of you a magical castle. Walk into the castle. Look at the beautiful rugs, the furniture, the paintings and the ceiling. To your right there is a room. Walk into the room. There is an antique mirror there. Look in the mirror. You see yourself as you are meant to be. You can do anything. You are confident and strong. You have vision and purpose. You are loving and enthusiastic. You feel emotionally stable and balanced. You know you are successful and are very special.

(Close your eyes for a moment and see how special you are.)

In the back of the room is a door. Walk to the door. There is a sign on the door. The sign says OPPORTUNITY. Open the door and walk into the room. There is a big, comfortable chair in the middle of the room. As you sit down in the chair you see all your problems come before you. It is different here. You know that all the problems are only situations in which you can grow. You are seeing your problems as opportunities. Watch as each problem presents itself and shows you the positive opportunities and how to resolve them. Whether the problems are of a physical, emotional, mental, or spiritual nature, watch as they appear before you one by one. Even if you can't see the opportunities, you know that you are absorbing the knowledge that you need. There is no effort and no judgment. Just watch and observe. Every time you have a problem, you see the opportunities.

(Close your eyes for a moment and watch.)

Now watch and feel positive energy as it comes into your body. You feel, know, and trust that you are becoming positive. There is no fear. No judgment. No expectation. Just a wonderful positive energy of this moment. You feel things shifting and you know that positive thought is becoming a part of your life. All the negative emotions just melt away. You feel centered and whole in body, mind, and spirit.

(Close your eyes for a moment and feel the positive energy.)

Keeping this positive energy with you, get up from the chair and walk out of the room. Walk outside of the castle. The sun is shining. The birds are singing joyously. You feel so positive and happy. You know you are able to conquer anything without effort. Look down at your feet and you can see your body asleep in the bed. You are drawn to your body and merge with it. The feeling of positive thought, love, peace, joy, and happiness will stay with you.

CHAPTER 5

Allergy

The Greek roots of the word allergy mean "abnormal response." Allergy occurs when normally harmless substances produce an abnormal response in the body. These substances include food, dust, pollen, mold, bacteria, plants, textiles, cosmetics, insect bites, animal fur, feathers, smoke, chemical pollutants, and drugs.

An allergen, sometimes called an antigen, is the cause of allergy; symptoms will vary. Some of the symptoms associated with allergy include watery eyes, runny nose, nasal congestion, sneezing, rash, hives, upset stomach, and breathing difficulties.

When the immune system mistakes a normally harmless substance for something harmful to the body, an allergic reaction occurs. The immune system detects this allergen or antigen and begins to manufacture an antibody, immunoglobulin E. The antibody then combines with the allergen and causes the release of active compounds, one of which is histamine. The histamine interacts with the blood vessels and mucous membranes, which then cause leakage, swelling, and congestion in the body.

Typically, when someone is first exposed to an allergen, no symptoms will occur. The immune system logs the initial contact of the allergen into its memory; when reexposure occurs, it reacts to produce an allergic reaction. Heredity plays a role in atopic allergies, in which there is no first exposure before the reaction. Some examples of atopic allergy are food allergies, asthma, eczema, and hay fever.

If you have identified an allergen, avoidance of the cause is the best prevention. For example, if you find out that you are allergic to a specific food, don't eat it. Of course, some allergens can't be avoided, so other steps need to be taken. Medical doctors and pharmacies use three types of medications: antihistamines, which block the histamine; anti-inflammatory agents, such as corticosteroids; and decongestants, which relieve congestion. Ask your pharmacist for the product insert from the medication's manufacturer and read about the possible side effects. You should be aware of what you are putting inside your body; you will be able to get additional facts from the product insert that can provide you with an intelligent choice. For example, decongestants can help for the short term, but have been proven to be counterproductive for the long term.

Homeopathic medicines stimulate the body to heal itself and can be used without side effects.

Allergy Relief Remedies

MENTAL ATTITUDE
Cause: rejecting the new.
Cure: act and say what's in your mind. Take time for you.

FOODS & DIET
Avoid: milk, wheat, beef, artificial colors and flavorings, food preservatives.
Good Foods: rice bran, vinegar, artichokes, garlic, olive oil, rose hips, cherries, papaya, lemon, squash, cashews, corn, pecans, soybeans, cabbage, and beans.

VITAMINS & SUPPLEMENTS
Vitamin C, calcium, magnesium, bromelain, bee pollen.

HERBS
Turmeric, quercetin, eyebright, goldenseal, echinacea, marigold, stinging nettle, ginkgo biloba.

AROMATHERAPY
Chamomile, melissa.

Self-hypnosis can lessen symptoms of allergy. One or more of the following scripts should be used in the morning, at dusk and right before you go to sleep. To optimize results, you may even want to try the scripts for asthma and other breathing problems, general illness, skin diseases, and stress.

ALLERGY SCRIPTS

THE BOAT
Intention: To eliminate allergy.

ind a comfortable place where you won't be disturbed, and sit in a comfortable chair. Now sit back and relax with both feet on the floor, and place your hands on the armrests of the chair or in your lap — whichever is comfortable for you.

Concentrate as you breathe deeply, letting the air come into your nose and out your mouth. Concentrate and breathe IN with the nose and OUT with the mouth. IN with the nose and OUT with the mouth. And IN with the nose and OUT with the mouth. Now let's concentrate on breathing OUT with the mouth and IN with the nose. And OUT with the mouth and IN with the nose. And OUT with the mouth and IN with the mouth.

Imagine you are very, very tiny. You are in a dark place in a very small boat. The boat is gently rocking and you feel safe and secure. As your eyes become accustomed to the darkness, you know you are inside your body. There is no fear, you are just filled with wonder and awe. In front of you there is a small point of white light. This light becomes brighter and brighter.

(Close your eyes for a moment and see this light.)

Look down in the bottom of the boat. There is a conductor's wand and a golden feather. Pick up the conductor's wand and point it at the light. The light moves. Wherever you move the wand, the light follows.

If you move the wand fast, the light gets brighter. If you move the wand slowly, the light gets dimmer. The white light is a healing light. You feel and know that this light can provide everything you need to help you heal your symptoms. You trust this light.

Look down at the bottom of the boat and pick up the golden feather. The feather is a magic feather and can move you and your boat to wherever your symptoms are occurring in your body. Watch as the feather gently guides your boat to wherever you have a symptom. You use your conductor's wand to light the way. Gently, smoothly going towards the place where your symptom is occurring in your body. It may be your eyes, your nose, your stomach, your lungs or your skin. Just relax and let the boat take you there, lighting the way with your wand.

(Close your eyes for a moment and feel the boat gliding to your symptom.)

When you are at the symptom site, you can see where the problem exists. It may be a different color or shape, but you can physically see the problem. You may not know the intricate details of the problem, but that does not matter. You have the healing light and you know that this light can heal the problem.

Raise your conductor's wand and direct the light towards your problem. Watch as the light glows brighter and brighter. Now watch as the problem begins to disappear. Shrinking away. Going away. You feel this. You know this. You trust that this is happening right now in this time, in this place. Watch, watch as the problem is just going away. Being healed by this wonderful white light. You feel your symptom just disappearing. Making you whole and healthy in your body. When the problem is gone and your symptom has disappeared, let the golden feather direct your boat to any other symptoms in your body. Heal each one with the white light. Feel each problem as it just disappears. Feel your symptoms disappear one by one by one.

(Close your eyes for a moment and go through your body, healing your symptoms.)

When you are done, place the feather at the bottom of the boat. The boat gently rocks you back and forth. Now place the conductor's wand in the bottom of the boat. Watch as the healing light fades in the distance. You know you have done very good work today. You feel happy, healthy and whole in body, mind, and spirit. This feeling will stay with you.

THE LAB
Intention: To eliminate allergy.

Find a comfortable place where you won't be disturbed, and sit in a comfortable chair. Now sit back and relax with both feet on the floor, and place your hands on the armrests of the chair or in your lap — whichever is comfortable for you.

Concentrate as you breathe deeply, letting the air come into your nose and out your mouth. Concentrate and breathe IN with the nose and OUT with the mouth. IN with the nose and OUT with the mouth. And IN with the nose and OUT with the mouth. Now let's concentrate on breathing OUT with the mouth and IN with the nose. And OUT with the mouth and IN with the nose. And OUT with the mouth and IN with the mouth.

Imagine you are in a scientific lab. The environment is clean and sterile. Everything is white. The light shines off the walls, the tables, and the floor. You are alone and feel very relaxed. Take a look around and notice all the things in the lab. So clean. So white. Look to your left. There is a small enclosed glass room with a bed in it. Walk over to the room and open the door. As you walk into the room, you smell your favorite smell. It makes you feel comfortable.

(Close your eyes for a moment and smell this wonderful smell.)

It is so comfortable here. Look at the bed; it is exactly the right size for you. It looks so inviting. Lie down on the bed and feel how comfortable it is. As you relax on the bed, take a look at the ceiling. There is an unusual light just above you. It is the most beautiful light you have ever seen. You feel different under this light. You feel strong, healthy, and filled with energy. The light coming from the fixture in the ceiling seems to dance around the room. Glinting. Sparkling. It is almost as if the light is joyful.

Feel the light surround your body. Feel it outline your body from the top of your head to the bottom of your feet. Surrounding you in brilliant bright white light. It's as if there is a halo around you. A halo of white healing, protective light. Feel the light go into your body. Feel the healing taking place. Every part of your body becoming healthy. You feel so safe and you know that your body is protected from anything that could make your immune system unstable. You feel so healthy. So protected.

(Close your eyes for a moment and feel the white light.)

Realizing that nothing negative can penetrate this light, get up from the bed. Notice how the halo of white light still surrounds you. You feel strong. You know you are protected. Wherever you move, this light moves with you. Surrounding you. Keeping you healthy.

Walk out of the glass room and take a look at the lab around you. So clean, so sterile. Look at your body and feel the light around you. This light will stay with you wherever you go. Keeping you healthy and safe. You are joyful and happy. This feeling will stay with you.

CHAPTER 6

Anger

In most cases, anger is an overreaction to a situation. A primary negative emotion, anger influences the entire person and how that person successfully reacts to his or her environment.

There are two types of anger: manifest anger and latent anger. Anger can be transient or chronic. If it is chronic, the anger is usually excessive and irrational. Impatience, constant hurrying, a sense of time urgency, self-centered behavior, verbal aggression, and hostility are some of the symptoms of manifest anger. Latent anger is a part of the subconscious mind and the person is usually unaware of it. Latent anger also plays a role in chronic depression.

The body reacts to anger by increasing respiratory rate, pulse rate, and blood to the muscles that move the body's bones. It also constricts the pupils of the eyes, and pumps out hormones from the adrenal gland.

Anger should be experienced and acknowledged, but should not inhabit the mind for any extended period of time. The best way to deal with anger is to recognize and deal with it in a positive way. Positive ways to deal with anger could include taking responsibility for behavior, negotiating with people, taking time out, and hitting a punching bag or a pillow. Remember not to drink alcohol and that negative emotional displays are not in your best interest.

The professional psychological approach usually deals with chronic anger in one of the following ways: The projection method helps one recognize how the anger is being used as an ego defense mechanism to deny the unconscious root of the anger. The behavioral approach explores practical ways to avoid people and situations that make one angry. The interpersonal approach focuses on developing communication skills to improve relationships with others. The cognitive approach helps to find and correct the distortion of your ideas about life and other people.

Anger is always negative and is a choice. By learning to acknowledge and then release anger, you open yourself up to change and renewal, and you can lead a happier life. Exercise can help get rid of anger and put you in a more positive mood. Try walking, biking, yoga, qi gong, or weight lifting to help dissipate the anger. Diet, supplements, herbs, aromatherapy, and meditation can help the physical and emotional levels.

Anger Relief Remedies

MENTAL ATTITUDE
Cause: incomplete understanding or unfulfilled desires.
Cure: release the past and go after your goals.

FOODS & DIET
Avoid: alcohol, sugar.
Good Foods: turnips, watercress, artichokes, oat bran, yogurt.

VITAMINS & SUPPLEMENTS
Multiple vitamin and mineral supplement, B complex, Vitamin C, coenzyme Q10, calcium, magnesium.

HERBS
Coriander, oat straw, kava, chamomile, peppermint, skullcap, vervain, linden flowers, gotu kola, hops.

AROMATHERAPY
Chamomile, melissa, ylang ylang, rose.

Self-hypnosis can aid anger. One or more of the following scripts should be used in the morning, at dusk, and right before you go to sleep. To optimize results, you may even want to try the scripts for depression, fear, guilt, and low self-esteem.

ANGER SCRIPTS

THE TELEVISION
Intention: To eliminate anger.

Find a comfortable place where you won't be disturbed, and sit in a comfortable chair. Now sit back and relax with both feet on the floor, and place your hands on the armrests of the chair or in your lap — whichever is comfortable for you.

Concentrate as you breathe deeply, letting the air come into your nose and out your mouth. Concentrate and breathe IN with the nose and OUT with the mouth. IN with the nose and OUT with the mouth. And IN with the nose and OUT with the mouth. Now let's concentrate on breathing OUT with the mouth and IN with the nose. And OUT with the mouth and IN with the nose. And OUT with the mouth and IN with the mouth.

Imagine you are sitting in a soft, comfortable chair with a very large TV screen in front of you. You are alone and trying to get centered. Watch as a light flickers on the TV screen. It seems to flicker very rapidly. It is flickering so fast that you cannot see the image. Now a red flashing light is seen on the screen. This red light is flicking faster and faster.

(Close your eyes for a moment and see the red light flashing.)

Watch as the red light turns to blue. The screen is getting centered. The blue color soothes you. It relaxes you. Feel how the blue color makes you feel calm. Let the blue light gently invade your mind until you start to feel centered.

(Close your eyes for a moment and see the blue light.)

Look at the screen and see yourself doing something you enjoy. See yourself taking your time and experiencing each moment. You don't have a care or worry in the world. See yourself feeling happy at what you are doing. You are elated and filled with joy.

A sense of love and well-being surrounds your mind and body. It permeates every cell of your being. Every cell, every fiber, every tissue, every muscle, every organ, every bone in your body is absorbing this love.

(Close your eyes for a moment and feel this love.)

You feel complete and whole. You are filled with positive thoughts. How happy and positive you feel. This feeling will stay with you.

OUT OF THE STORM
Intention: To eliminate anger.

Find a comfortable place where you won't be disturbed, and sit in a comfortable chair. Now sit back and relax with both feet on the floor, and place your hands on the armrests of the chair or in your lap — whichever is comfortable for you.

Concentrate as you breathe deeply, letting the air come into your nose and out your mouth. Concentrate and breathe IN with the nose and OUT with the mouth. IN with the nose and OUT with the mouth. And IN with the nose and OUT with the mouth. Now let's concentrate on breathing OUT with the mouth and IN with the nose. And OUT with the mouth and IN with the nose. And OUT with the mouth and IN with the mouth.

Imagine you are walking down a path in the woods. You are alone. You are walking at your own pace. Look at the trees around you. See the colors of the leaves. Hear the leaves rustling around you as you walk by the trees. Feel the wind around you. Stop for a moment and look up at the sky. There are dark clouds overhead and it is getting darker. You know that these are thunderclouds. Look at these clouds as they gather over you. Feel the storm brewing in the sky above you. The wind is blowing harder. The clouds are getting bigger and darker. Smell the air and feel it grow closer around you.

You start to hear the roll of thunder. Watch as a flash of lightning reaches out across the sky. Watch as the sky lights up. Feel the power of the lightning. Hear the rolls of thunder booming all around you. Loud and sharp. Feel the power of the thunder. This is a very big storm.

(Close your eyes for a moment and see the storm.)

Drops of rain are now starting to fall. The drops of rain are falling on top of you. Feel them on your hair, your arms, your clothes. Look down the path. A short distance away, you see a house. Walk towards the house as the rain falls harder and harder. The house has a covered porch. Walk onto the porch and turn around. Watch as the rain continues to pour down harder and harder. Protected on the porch, see the torrents of rain fall on the ground. Hear the thunder roll across the sky. See the lightning continue to flash.

(Close your eyes for a moment and see the storm.)

Turn towards the door of the house and open it. This is your special place. All the things in the house are as you have always wanted them. The color of the carpet is your favorite color. The room is cozy and warm. Look around the room and to the left you see a fireplace with a comfortable chair in front of it. Sit down in the chair, it is exactly right for you. There is a blazing fire in the fireplace. The flames are filled with colors. Feel the fire dry your clothes as you sit comfortably in the chair. You feel warm and protected from the storm outside. Feel the contentment start to seep into your body. Feel how centered and calm you are becoming.

(Close your eyes for a moment and feel the peace.)

You are out of the storm. You are safe. Feel the rays of happiness start to infiltrate your body making you whole and at peace right now. When you are ready, turn and look out the window. See the sun's rays coming through the window and making bright patterns on the floor. Hear the birds singing outside. You smile and are happy. You are centered and at peace. This feeling will stay with you.

CHAPTER 7

Anxiety

Anxiety is an unpleasant emotion generated within yourself. It gives you a vague, unspecified feeling that harm is going to come to you in some way. You can't really be specific that the harm is going to come; you may not even know where it will come from, but you have the feeling anyway. Extreme forms of anxiety are called panic attacks.

The powerful feelings of anxiety can involve some or all of these physical symptoms: a rapid heartbeat, body tremors, sweating, difficulty in breathing, dry mouth, chest tightness, dizziness, insomnia, fatigue, cramps, loss of appetite, sweaty palms, nausea, or diarrhea. The physical symptoms are real. There may even be some mental symptoms that occur, including changes in your sex drive, inability to concentrate, disorganized behavior, and even the inability to do more than one thing at one time.

In psychology there are several theories as to the cause of anxiety. Learning theory considers anxiety a reaction to pain, so therapists suggest staying away from the source of the pain. Cognitive theory focuses on finding the cause of the problem; therapists suggest using positive self-talk to combat anxiety. Physiological theory suggests giving drugs to combat anxiety. Sometimes there is no other alternative, but most drugs cause side effects. Many of the "designer" drugs given for anxiety have side effects that can create anxiety. Ask your pharmacist for the insert that the manufacturer includes with the drugs and read it. Consider the possible side effects and the fact that some of these drugs sometimes stay in the body for years after you stop taking them; then make your decision as to whether this is the type of treatment you want or need.

Psychoanalytic theory states that two types of anxiety are recognized: 1) anxiety resulting from trauma and 2) signal anxiety, which is in effect when someone is trying to protect himself from anxiety resulting from trauma.

No matter what the theory, anxiety relates to a future time and is usually about a future situation. It also comes from scattered attention and lack of focus. It is the unknown that causes apprehension and anxiousness. Living in the moment can help stop anxiety. We deceive ourselves into thinking we can control, manipulate, or modify the future. In actuality, there are so many variables that we really can't see all the possibilities that can occur. In fact, worrying or being anxious causes more anxiety and may cause missing a moment that could be truly valuable.

There is a paradox to anxiety: the more you anticipate what's going to happen, the more anxious you become. To eliminate anxiety, becoming quiet and allowing things to happen works better than being anxious about what might happen. Learn to give your full attention to everything you do in the moment. By letting go of the anxiety, you conquer it. Living in the moment does help.

Since anxiety is based on the fear of a future outcome, you can learn to cope with this fear by using positive thought. Remember: you are what you think! Negative emotions bring negative results. Positive emotions bring positive results, so learn to laugh at the outcome and think positive!

Focusing on the breath and breathing is very important when you become anxious. Breathing slowly and deeply activates the vagus nerve, which is the major quieting nerve of the body. This nerve helps to calm you down automatically, so when you become anxious, deep breathing can help.

To prevent anxiety and center yourself, several exercise programs that include breath work are helpful — for example, tai chi, yoga, and qi gong.

Anxiety Relief Remedies

MENTAL ATTITUDE
Cause: unsettled and scattered attention.
Cure: positive thought and living in the moment.

FOODS & DIET
Avoid: sugar, caffeine, nicotine, artificial flavorings, colors and preservatives.
Good Foods: increase protein foods, oat bran, yogurt, turnips, and watercress.

VITAMINS & SUPPLEMENTS
Vitamin C, A, B12, B1, niacin; inositol, chromium, manganese, calcium, magnesium, phosphorus and potassium.

HERBS
St. John's wort, vervain, linden flowers, kava, oat straw, skullcap, lemon balm, valerian, passionflower, hops, bilberry, and wood betony.

AROMATHERAPY
Rose, marjoram, sandalwood, geranium, neroli, lavender, melissa, bergamot and jasmine.

Self-hypnosis is a very positive way to help you conquer anxiety. The following scripts should be used in the morning and at night for at least six weeks. When you start to become anxious during the day, focus on the breath and breathing. If you have time during the day, do a self-hypnosis script. To optimize results, you may even want to combine the anxiety scripts with the ones for stress.

ANXIETY SCRIPTS

THE PARADE
Intention: To eliminate anxiety.

Find a comfortable place where you won't be disturbed, and sit in a comfortable chair. Now sit back and relax with both feet on the floor, and place your hands on the armrests of the chair or in your lap — whichever is comfortable for you.

Concentrate as you breathe deeply, letting the air come into your nose and out your mouth. Concentrate and breathe IN with the nose and OUT with the mouth. IN with the nose and OUT with the mouth. And IN with the nose and OUT with the mouth. Now let's concentrate on breathing OUT with the mouth and IN with the nose. And OUT with the mouth and IN with the nose. And OUT with the mouth and IN with the mouth.

Imagine yourself walking in a parade. People are all around you. There is a band playing. Listen to the music. Hear the drums beat. Look at the people and how they are dressed. Look over to your right and see the people watching the parade as it goes by. See the looks of expectation on their faces, the colors, the flags.

(Close your eyes for a moment and see the people.)

Look to your left and see the children. See the balloons they are holding, the ice cream cones. Look at their smiling faces. Hear their laughter.

(Close your eyes for a moment and see the children.)

Look over your shoulder to the back of you. See all the people marching behind you. See the baton twirlers. Listen to the band's music.

Now look in front of you. See how the street curves out of sight before you. *Take a deep breath and exhale.* Look even closer in front of you and see how narrow the street becomes. Watch as the marchers ahead of you start to stop and are just marching in time. *Take a deep breath and exhale.* Notice the parade is backing up. *Take a deep breath and exhale.* The more you march to the front, the more and more backed up the way in front of you becomes. Look to the back of you. Hear and watch as the marchers keep getting closer and closer.

(Close your eyes for a moment and feel the closeness.)

Look to your left. See an opening in the crowd. Walk towards this opening. Look to your right side and see how few people are really around you. Keep walking through the opening until you find your-self in the most beautiful garden you have ever seen. There is no one here but you. It feels safe and you know that this is your special pri-vate place. Breathe in deeply and smell the flowers. Hear the birds sing. Feel the sun warming your body. The sun's rays so warm, so comforting.

(Close your eyes for a moment and see the garden.)

You feel centered. You feel calm. You feel peace.

Look down at your body and see how calm it is. How centered you feel. Breathing evenly and smoothly. Feel the tension being drawn away as the sun warms your body. Feeling so secure. Without a worry in the world. Knowing everything is taken care of. You feel happy.

(Close your eyes for a moment and feel the calmness.)

Remember how you feel now, in this time, in this place. This feeling will stay with you.

THE BLUE LIGHT
Intention: To eliminate anxiety.

Find a comfortable place where you won't be disturbed, and sit in a comfortable chair. Now sit back and relax with both feet on the floor, and place your hands on the armrests of the chair or in your lap — whichever is comfortable for you.

Concentrate as you breathe deeply, letting the air come into your nose and out your mouth. Concentrate and breathe IN with the nose and OUT with the mouth. IN with the nose and OUT with the mouth. And IN with the nose and OUT with the mouth. Now let's concentrate on breathing OUT with the mouth and IN with the nose. And OUT with the mouth and IN with the nose. And OUT with the mouth and IN with the mouth.

Imagine that you are standing in a room. There is activity all around you. Look up over your head. See an electric blue light. It is the most beautiful blue light you have ever seen. Look at it shine . . . sparkle . . . glimmer. Watch as this blue light starts to surround the right side of your body. Watch as it forms an outline around you. It feels so safe. It feels so comfortable.

(Close your eyes for a moment and feel this blue light.)

You feel this blue light absorbing all the stress, all the tension from your body. Watch as it goes down the right side of your body down to your right foot. Watch and feel all the stress and all the tension being absorbed by this blue light as it goes underneath your foot and outlines your inner right leg. See the light go down your inner left leg and under your left foot. So soothing. So comforting. Now feel the light go up your left leg and up your torso, your arm, your shoulder. Outlining the body. Drawing away all the tension all the stress. Making you feel so calm, so centered.

(Close your eyes for a moment and see and feel the blue light.)

Watch as this blue light attaches to where it started. Fully outlining the body. Feel the glow of the light around you. Feel it absorbing any stress or tension that is left in your body. Making you feel calm and safe right here, in this time, in this place. You feel peaceful in this blue light. You are centered. This is your protective light. You are safe within this light. You can imagine this light whenever you need it. Whenever you feel anxious, this blue light will surround your body. Absorbing the tension. Absorbing the stress. Making you feel centered and safe. This feeling will stay with you.

CHAPTER 8

Arthritis

About 50 million Americans suffer from arthritis. Arthritis is defined as joint inflammation and affects the joints, connective tissue, and support tissue. Over 100 rheumatic diseases may be diagnosed as arthritis. However, true arthritis is either osteoarthritis or rheumatoid arthritis.

Osteoarthritis typically starts after the age of 40 and progresses gradually. This type of arthritis is caused by the wear and tear placed on the cartilage around the joints. The cartilage, once smooth, becomes rough, and calcium deposits or spurs then form on the joints. The spurs then make contact with the bone and nerves, which results in stiffness and pain. In addition, the tissues around the joint and bone normally provide an insulating fluid that cushions the contact between the joints and the bone. With osteoarthritis, this fluid becomes thick; that is what makes movement painful and difficult. Osteoarthritis may produce limited joint mobility, inflammation, and enlargement of the joint. Osteoarthritis affects individual joints, which may make popping and clicking noises.

Rheumatoid arthritis is a chronic inflammation, which causes stiffness, swelling, pain, and deformity to muscles and joints. An autoimmune disorder, rheumatoid arthritis frequently occurs in people under 40 years of age. The problem occurs when the immune system improperly identifies the synovial membrane (which secretes the lubricating fluid around the joints) as harmful to the body. The immune system then attacks the synovial membrane, resulting in inflammation and sometimes damaging or destroying the cartilage and tissue surrounding the joint. The body replaces the tissue that is damaged or destroyed with scar tissue. This scar tissue may cause the bones to fuse together. Rheumatoid arthritis affects all synovial joints, which tend to make a crackling sound.

The causes of arthritis may be tied to consumption of processed foods; environmental toxins; nutritional deficiencies; food allergies; obesity; or bacterial, fungal, or viral infection. There are many prescription drugs available on the market. Ask your pharmacist to let you see the insert to explore the side effects of a drug before making a decision on using it. Changing to a low-fat, high-fiber, mostly vegetarian diet and regular exercise, such walking, yoga, tai chi, or qi gong may help. Noninvasive homeopathic remedies and acupuncture are excellent methods to use to reduce the pain of arthritis.

Arthritis Relief Remedies

MENTAL ATTITUDE

Cause: anger and mental restriction.
Cure: positive thoughts like: I can, I will, I am.

FOODS & DIET

Avoid: sugar, caffeine, nicotine, alcohol, artificial flavorings, colors, preservatives, processed foods, animal fats, eggplant, green peppers, potatoes, tomatoes.

Good Foods: grapefruit, garlic, grapes, pineapple, almonds, kiwi fruit, horseradish, lentils, salmon, sardines, watercress, walnuts, broccoli, corn, cashews, guavas, cherries, green onions, tuna, lime.

VITAMINS & SUPPLEMENTS

Multivitamin and mineral supplement with whole foods and enzymes, Vitamin C, K, E, D, B complex, folic acid, manganese, boron, EPA (eicosapentaenoic acid) fish oil, coenzyme Q10, bromelain, SOD (superoxide desmutase), germanium, chondroitin, glucosamine sulfate.

HERBS

Yucca, angelica, willow, devil's claw, celery seed, ginger, turmeric, basil.

AROMATHERAPY

Eucalyptus, rosemary, juniper, benzoin, and lavender.

The following scripts should be used in the morning and at night for at least six weeks. To optimize results, you may even want to try the scripts for general illness, pain, and stress.

ARTHRITIS SCRIPTS

THE HEALING MUD
Intention: To relieve arthritis pain.

Find a comfortable place where you won't be disturbed, and sit in a comfortable chair. Now sit back and relax with both feet on the floor, and place your hands on the armrests of the chair or in your lap — whichever is comfortable for you.

Concentrate as you breathe deeply, letting the air come into your nose and out your mouth. Concentrate and breathe IN with the nose and OUT with the mouth. IN with the nose and OUT with the mouth. And IN with the nose and OUT with the mouth. Now let's concentrate on breathing OUT with the mouth and IN with the nose. And OUT with the mouth and IN with the nose. And OUT with the mouth and IN with the mouth.

Imagine that you are in a meadow. The sun is warm and shining brightly. The sky is blue and cloudless. It is a perfect day. Look at the green grass, the flowers, and the trees that surround the meadow. Smell the balmy air.

Look to your right. There is a pool of water shining in the sun. Look at the clean, clear water sparkling in the sun. It is so tranquil and serene here. You know that this water is special. You are alone and this is your private place. No one can enter here. Take off your clothes and lay them on the grass by the pond. The temperature is just right for you. Step into the water and feel how warm it is as it reaches your feet and ankles. Wade into the water, find a comfortable spot, and sit down. It is not deep. Feel the water embrace your thighs, your stomach, your shoulders and your neck. Relaxing in this wonderful water, you feel so relaxed.

(Close your eyes for a moment and feel how relaxed you are.)

Look down and see the soft white mud. Touch the mud and feel how soothing it is. Feel the tension just float away as you relax in the water. You are so comfortable. Now feel yourself sinking into the mud. Feel the mud surround each joint and muscle of your body. It is so soothing. Feel the mud start to go into your body, surrounding the muscles, the bones and joints. Watch the mud as it draws the toxins from around your muscles, your bones and your joints.

(Close your eyes for a moment and feel the mud taking out the toxins.)

Imagine the mud drawing away the pain. Absorbing the pain and taking it away from the body. How good this feels. Now feel the warm mud absorbing the calcium deposits that are on your cartilage and tissues. Imagine the white healing mud drawing and absorbing the pain, making your joints free and limber. Healing you in this time, in this place right now.

(Close your eyes for a moment and feel the healing.)

Feel the pain drain away in the mud. Relax in the mud and know you are healing. When you are ready, watch as the mud comes out of your body the same way it went in. Taking with it all the pain, all the inflammation.

Stand up in the water and wash the remaining mud off your body. Step out of the pond and lie down on the soft green grass, and look up at the sky. Feel the sun dry you off. Feel the rays of the sun on your body. Feel the warm tones of blue and green light coming from the sun. This light surrounds each joint and muscle, healing any residual pain that is left inside your body.

(Close your eyes for a moment and feel this light.)

Your body is free from pain. Your joints are limber and supple. Stretch them and see how good it feels. When you are done, stand up and put your clothes back on. You are comfortable, happy and at peace. This feeling will stay with you.

OUT IN SPACE
Intention: To relieve arthritis pain.

Find a comfortable place where you won't be disturbed, and sit in a comfortable chair. Now sit back and relax with both feet on the floor, and place your hands on the armrests of the chair or in your lap — whichever is comfortable for you.

Concentrate as you breathe deeply, letting the air come into your nose and out your mouth. Concentrate and breathe IN with the nose and OUT with the mouth. IN with the nose and OUT with the mouth. And IN with the nose and OUT with the mouth. Now let's concentrate on breathing OUT with the mouth and IN with the nose. And

OUT with the mouth and IN with the nose. And OUT with the mouth and IN with the mouth.

Imagine you are floating in space. The bright stars are all around you. You feel free and calm without a care or worry in the world. Your body is weightless and there is no strain, tension or pain in any part of your body. You just feel comfortable and happy.

(Close your eyes for a moment and feel the weightlessness.)

Look at the stars around you. The light is so bright and warm. It feels so wonderful. Watch as the stars send beams of light to your joints and muscles. Feel this light permeate your tissues, muscles, bones, and joints. Warming them. Soothing them. This magic starlight makes your joints move so easily, without pain or stiffness. The starlight is absorbing all the pain, the inflammation, and any discomfort. One by one they just disappear as you just float in space without a care or worry in the world.

(Close your eyes for a moment and feel the healing.)

Watch as the starlight comes out of your body the same way it went in. Feeling very relaxed and pain-free, move your joints. How wonderful to move them without stiffness or pain. There is no discomfort. You just float in space feeling very, very relaxed. What wonderful starlight this is. As you look at the stars twinkling, you feel very happy and peaceful. Float as long as you like. This feeling will stay with you.

CHAPTER 9

Asthma and Other Breathing Problems

Asthma and breathing problems can be caused by emotional stress, environmental factors, allergies, or viral respiratory disease. Asthma results in obstruction of the lung's bronchii or airways. Muscle spasms surrounding the bronchii constrict, impeding the exhalation of stale air from the lungs. Over time, asthma can affect the lung tissue's capacity to stretch. This could lead to serious breathing problems. Symptoms of asthma can include difficulty in breathing, wheezing, coughing, and a feeling of chest tightness.

Allergens provoke asthma attacks. Allergens are substances that the immune system interprets as harmful to the body. The immune system reacts by producing antibodies, which combine with the allergen to release histamine. The histamine interacts with the mucous membranes and blood vessels, which causes swelling and congestion. Common allergens include: animal dander, fumes, mold, feathers, chemicals, and tobacco smoke. Asthma attacks and breathing problems also can be caused by adrenal disorders, humidity, low blood sugar, temperature changes, fear, anxiety, and stress.

People with asthma may be sensitive to sulfites used as food additives. Many over-the-counter and prescription drugs can produce side effects that constrict the bronchii muscles. Food allergies can trigger asthmatic reactions. Some common culprits are dairy products, pork, white sugar, wheat, food colorings, MSG (monosodium glutamate), alfalfa, corn, processed foods, beets, and cola drinks.

A proper diet and regular exercise is beneficial. Ionizing air purifiers eliminate dust, mold, bacteria, pollen, and pollutants from the air. Meditation, yoga, and other techniques can help reduce stress, which is always beneficial.

Asthma Relief Remedies

MENTAL ATTITUDE
Cause: fear and denial of oneself.
Cure: develop a plan of what you want to say, feel, or do.

FOODS & DIET
Avoid: sugar, artificial flavorings, colors, preservatives, beans, broccoli, cauliflower, cabbage, ice cream, cold liquids, and processed foods.
Good Foods: turnips, pumpkin, radishes, chicken, kelp, grapefruit, horseradish, onions, squash.

VITAMINS & SUPPLEMENTS
Multivitamin and mineral supplement with whole foods and enzymes, Vitamin C, A, B complex, bioflavonoids, beta carotene, coenzyme Q10, calcium, magnesium, L-cysteine, quercetin, and bee pollen.

HERBS
Pau d'arco, ginkgo biloba, lobelia, chamomile, eucalyptus, horehound, kava, cowslip, thyme, garlic, echinacea, and evening primrose oil.

AROMATHERAPY
Eucalyptus, hyssop, cypress, benzoin, lavender, melissa, and marjoram.

The following scripts should be used in the morning and at night for at least six weeks. To optimize results, you may even want to try the scripts for allergy, general illness, and stress.

ASTHMA & BREATHING PROBLEM SCRIPTS

THE EUCALYPTUS GROVE
Intention: To relieve asthma and breathing problems.

Find a comfortable place where you won't be disturbed, and sit in a comfortable chair. Now sit back and relax with both feet on the floor, and place your hands on the armrests of the chair or in your lap — whichever is comfortable for you.

Concentrate as you breathe deeply, letting the air come into your nose and out your mouth. Concentrate and breathe IN with the nose and OUT with the mouth. IN with the nose and OUT with the mouth. And IN with the nose and OUT with the mouth. Now let's concentrate on breathing OUT with the mouth and IN with the nose. And

OUT with the mouth and IN with the nose. And OUT with the mouth and IN with the mouth.

Imagine you are walking down a path in the woods. Listen to the birds sing. See and smell the wildflowers along the path. What bright colors they are. The sky is blue and the sun is shining. The temperature is just right for you. Watch as the clouds move slowly in the sky. How relaxed you are. Look to your right. You see a grove of eucalyptus trees. The trees are very old and tall. The barks of the trees are made of silver and they have many leaves. The leaves are made of very thin gold and they sparkle as the sun hits them.

(Close your eyes for a moment and picture the trees.)

Step off the path and walk towards the trees. As you get nearer, you begin to smell the odor of eucalyptus. It is fresh and pungent. Take a deep breath and smell this odor. Now walk into the center of the trees. The grass is soft beneath your feet and the sun's rays make beautiful patterns as they shine off the golden leaves of the trees. You feel peaceful and calm as you breathe in the beauty around you. Raise your hands over your head and breathe in the odor of the trees. Feel the smell enter into your nose. Feel the odor fill your nose. Watch as the odor becomes a golden light. The golden light feels wonderful and comforting. Feel the light go down your nasal passages. As the light passes through, it is absorbing all the congestion.

(Close your eyes for a moment and breathe in this golden light.)

Now see the golden light turn gray at its center as it absorbs the congestion within itself. See and feel the golden light get brighter around the gray as it captures the congestion so it cannot escape. Watch and feel the golden light cleansing each area it passes on its way to the lungs. Breathing deeper and deeper, without pain just feeling so very, very relaxed. Now watch and feel the golden light enter the lungs. As the light passes into the lungs, each cell is cleansed by the light. Any congestion is absorbed by the light. The light soothing each area as it fills the lungs. Cleaning out the infection, healing each cell as it passes.

(Close your eyes for a moment and feel the light healing the lungs.)

Feel the light soothing and healing you. You are so calm and relaxed. All the tension just melts away from your body as you continue to breathe in the golden light. Now exhale and imagine the golden light coming out of your lungs and being expelled from your nose. You know that golden light is taking all the congestion away from your body. Keep breathing in and out until all the golden light is gone. Look up at the trees. The leaves are of thin gold tinkling in the wind. You can smell the eucalyptus. Take a breath and feel the air flow freely. You are happy and content. You will keep this feeling with you.

THE HEALING BREATH
Intention: To relieve asthma and breathing problems.

Find a comfortable place where you won't be disturbed, and sit in a comfortable chair. Now sit back and relax with both feet on the floor, and place your hands on the armrests of the chair or in your lap — whichever is comfortable for you.

Concentrate as you breathe deeply, letting the air come into your nose and out your mouth. Concentrate and breathe IN with the nose and OUT with the mouth. IN with the nose and OUT with the mouth. And IN with the nose and OUT with the mouth. Now let's concentrate on breathing OUT with the mouth and IN with the nose. And OUT with the mouth and IN with the nose. And OUT with the mouth and IN with the mouth.

Imagine you are standing in a room all alone. You are wearing comfortable clothing and the only thing in the room is a floor-to-ceiling mirror. Look at yourself in the mirror. You are relaxed and centered. Take a deep breath and imagine this breath going to any trouble spot in your body. Imagine the breath healing any problem spot as you breathe in and out very deeply and very methodically. With each breath, a trouble spot disappears. Continue breathing in and out until you feel all the trouble spots are gone.

(Close your eyes for a moment and feel the breath heal you.)

Now feel how free and easy you are breathing. You feel very relaxed and calm. Breathe in with your healing breath and watch as the breath goes into your mind. You feel the breath absorbing any stress and any negative emotion. As you breathe out, this stress and emotion comes out of your mind and out of your body. Feel the breath go to any area of your mind that needs healing. Feel the breath do its work.

(Close your eyes for a moment and feel the healing.)

Now take a deep breath and feel the positive energy fill your body. This feeling will stay with you.

CHAPTER 10

Backache

Backache can come from various sources, including: spinal degeneration; a slipped or herniated disk; constipation; arthritis; rheumatism; and tendon, ligament, bone, muscle, kidney, prostate, bladder, and pelvic problems.

The most common cause of backache is strain and sprain of the muscles, tendons, and ligaments supporting the back. Muscle strain and sprain affects the erector spinae muscles, which are the muscles that surround the spinal column. Tendon and ligament strain and sprain usually affect the lower sacroiliac back area. This area is located on the two sides of the pelvic area and includes a triangular bone located in the middle called the sacrum. Improper lifting, sitting, and posture are among the most common causes of backache.

Another common cause of backache is subluxation of the spinal vertebrae or sacroiliac joint. A subluxation is a partial dislocation or an alteration in the range of motion of the individual vertebra caused by injury or chronic improper standing, sitting, or lying down postures.

Backache can also be caused by improper footwear, sleeping on a soft mattress, calcium deficiencies, or stress and emotional problems.

When placed under strain, muscles contract. This muscle contraction produces two types of acids: lactic and pyruvic. If high levels of these acids are produced and are present in the muscles, irritation starts to occur. This irritation interferes with the normal electrical impulses in the tissue, which then turns the irritation into pain.

Proper posture when standing and sitting can help prevent and alleviate backache. A chair that supports the lower spine is best used for prolonged sitting. To avoid sprain and strain to the back when lifting heavy objects, bend your knees, use your leg muscles, and keep the article you are lifting close to your body. Sometimes the body is dehydrated. If you drink two glasses of water when pain hits, it may provide relief. Using ice packs on an injury within the first 48 hours may provide relief. After the initial 48 hours, a warm bath can help to relieve backache. Exercise such as yoga, bicycling, walking, rowing, and swimming can strengthen the abdominal muscles to help support the back. Meditation and other relaxation techniques have been shown to benefit backache. Chiropractic care is considered by many to be the treatment of choice for back problems.

Backache Relief Remedies

MENTAL ATTITUDE
Cause: inflexibility to change.
Cure: accept and create change each day.

FOODS & DIET
Avoid: sugar, alcohol, caffeine, nicotine, artificial flavorings, colors, preservatives.
Good Foods: purified water, swordfish, halibut, papaya, almonds, sardines, salmon.

VITAMINS & SUPPLEMENTS
Multivitamin and mineral supplement with whole foods and enzymes, Vitamin C, D, A, E, B12, silica, zinc, copper, born, calcium, magnesium, manganese.

HERBS
White willow bark, oat straw, horsetail, slippery elm, alfalfa, arnica ointment.

AROMATHERAPY
Lavender, chamomile, rose, eucalyptus.

The following scripts should be used in the morning and at night for at least six weeks. To optimize results, you may even want to try the scripts for pain, general illness, and stress.

BACKACHE SCRIPTS

THE SOLAR RAYS
Intention: To relieve backache pain.

Find a comfortable place where you won't be disturbed, and sit in a comfortable chair. Now sit back and relax with both feet on the floor, and place your hands on the armrests of the chair or in your lap — whichever is comfortable for you.

Concentrate as you breathe deeply, letting the air come into your nose and out your mouth. Concentrate and breathe IN with the nose and OUT with the mouth. IN with the nose and OUT with the mouth. And IN with the nose and OUT with the mouth. Now let's concentrate on breathing OUT with the mouth and IN with the nose. And OUT with the mouth and IN with the nose. And OUT with the mouth and IN with the mouth.

Imagine you are at the beach. You hear the waves gently rolling into shore. The sky is a beautiful shade of blue. You are lying on your stomach, just relaxing in the sun. You can feel the sun warming your legs, your back, your shoulders. The heat is so softly warm, at exactly the right temperature for you.

(Close your eyes for a moment and feel the sun.)

As you lie in the sun, without a care or worry in the world, feel how the sun's rays go into your back in exactly the places that you feel any pain or aches.

As the sun's rays go into your back, feel them absorbing all the pain. Feel the pain just flowing away from your back and into the rays. Softly, gently absorbing all the pain, all the stress in your back. You feel all your pain release and going away from your body.

(Close your eyes for a moment and feel the pain leave your body.)

Now feel the sun's rays gently shifting your body. All the bones in your back come into alignment. Each disk slipping into its proper place, without pain, without effort. Feel the sun's rays warm and soothing in your back as this shifting takes place. Now feel all your tendons, all your bones, all your muscles and all your joints as they gently shift back into alignment, one by one by one. Relieving any pain right now in this time, in this place.

(Close your eyes for a moment and feel your back come into alignment.)

Feel how the golden light of the sun enters your body and finds all the sources of your backache. No matter what part of the body is causing your pain, feel how the golden light of the sun finds the source of the pain. Now feel how the golden rays start healing all the sources of your problem. Balancing the acids, taking away all the irritation deep inside your body.

(Close your eyes for a moment and feel the balancing of your body.)

You know you are healing. You feel the sun's golden rays making your body so very, very relaxed. Feeling stress-free. Feeling happy as all the pain leaves your body. Feel how relaxed you are as every care, every worry leaves your body. Now watch as the sun's rays come out of your body the same way they went in.

You feel pain-free and so very relaxed. You feel very happy and joyful. This feeling will stay with you.

THE GENTLE HANDS
Intention: To relieve backache pain.

Find a comfortable place where you won't be disturbed, and sit in a comfortable chair. Now sit back and relax with both feet on the floor, and place your hands on the armrests of the chair or in your lap — whichever is comfortable for you.

Concentrate as you breathe deeply, letting the air come into your nose and out your mouth. Concentrate and breathe IN with the nose and OUT with the mouth. IN with the nose and OUT with the mouth. And IN with the nose and OUT with the mouth. Now let's concentrate on breathing OUT with the mouth and IN with the nose. And OUT with the mouth and IN with the nose. And OUT with the mouth and IN with the mouth.

Imagine you are in a most comfortable room. You are lying on your stomach on a massage table. Feel how relaxed you are. Smell the exotic oils in the air. Hear the soft melodious music. The temperature in the room is exactly right for you. You are so very, very relaxed.

(Close your eyes for a moment and feel how relaxed you are.)

Watch as several tiny hands appear in the air above your back. You somehow know that these are magic hands that are going to help you. Watch as the hands go to each spot on your back that has pain. Feel the hands gently massaging your back all at the same time. These hands are soothing your back. Feel the healing heat come from the palms of each hand. Now feel the hands massaging you gently, yet so effectively. The heat from the hands absorbs the pain and discomfort in your back. Feel how the stress is leaving your body. Feel the tension leaving your body. Every muscle, every tendon, every ligament and every bone in your body becomes relaxed.

(Close your eyes for a moment and feel how relaxed you are.)

Now feel the hands working together, adjusting your body. The hands are aligning each area of your body and putting everything in exactly the right place for you.

Relief floods your body. Peace enters your mind, as the gentle, effective healing hands make your body the best it can be. Feel the last remnants of pain leaving your body. You are more relaxed than you have ever known yourself to be. Allow the hands to work on your body as long as you need.

(Close your eyes for a moment and feel the healing taking place.)

When you are done, watch as the hands disappear. This is your private place that you can come back to whenever you need to. Feeling pain-free, relaxed, and happy you know this feeling will stay with you.

CHAPTER 11

Breast Cancer

The breast contains lymphatic vessels, milk ducts, lobes, and fatty tissue. In fact, the breast is mainly a round mass of glandular tissue with fifteen to twenty lobes. Each lobe has a duct that leads to an opening in the nipple. The framework of the breast is composed of connective tissue with a ligament layer beneath the breast, which provides firmness.

Most breast lumps are cysts and fibroid masses that are not cancerous. Cancerous tumors and lumps never go away. They are firm, usually pain-free, and can appear in any part of the breast. A biopsy may be needed to determine if a lump is cancerous. Some of the symptoms of breast cancer are: thickening of the breast; lumps; and redness, soreness, or itchiness of the nipple.

There are several kinds of breast cancer. They are categorized by the site where the cancer cells originated and the area of the breast in which they are located. These are: Paget's disease of the nipple, lobular carcinoma (breast lobe cancer), in situ (localized) breast duct cancer, intraductal carcinoma, ductal carcinoma (invasive milk duct cancer), inflammatory carcinoma (lymphatic/duct/blood vessel cancer), and several other uncommon types.

Cancer is unrestrained cell growth. Heredity, estrogen, and environmental factors seem to be the main cause of breast cancer. Estrogen promotes cellular growth in the breast. Environmental factors such as pesticides, chemicals, radiation, and silicone implants have been linked to breast cancer. There is an increased risk for breast cancer among women who are childless; are in menopause; started menstruating before 9 years of age; had a child after 40 years of age; consume large amounts of caffeine, alcohol and sugar; have diabetes; use oral contraceptives; and eat high-fat diets.

Traditional medical treatment of breast cancer includes surgery, radiation, chemotherapy, and chemotherapy plus bone marrow treatment. Please check out each treatment thoroughly and know the risks. Before you make a decision: Research! Research! Research! Ask questions and get the answers.

Natural health care treatments include nontoxic plant or human cell medications, immune system treatments, herbal remedies, nutritional diet therapies, detoxification therapies, ozone and oxygen therapies, and mind-body therapies.

Breast Cancer Relief Remedies

MENTAL ATTITUDE

Cause: resistance to feminine identity.
Cure: embrace the feminine self.

FOODS & DIET

Avoid: meat, processed food, animal and vegetable oils, white flour, sugar, salt, alcohol, caffeine, drugs, nicotine, artificial flavorings, colors, preservatives.

Good Foods: low-fat, high-fiber, mostly vegetarian diet; whole grains, fruits, vegetables, spinach, cabbage, red and green peppers, turnips, strawberries, filberts, horseradish, yogurt, maitake mushrooms, cashews, tomatoes, broccoli, avocados, salt water fish, brown rice, corn, alfalfa, soybeans, kelp, and onions.

VITAMINS & SUPPLEMENTS

Multivitamin and mineral supplement with whole foods and enzymes, Vitamin C, A, E, B12, B6, bioflavonoids, choline, germanium, SOD (superoxide desmutase), selenium, shark cartilage, betaine hydrochloric acid, acidophilus, coenzyme Q10.

HERBS

Cumin, garlic, evening primrose oil, red clover, Essiac tea, green tea.

AROMATHERAPY

Eucalyptus, hyssop, bergamot, geranium.

The following script should be used in the morning and at night for at least six weeks. To optimize results, you may even want to try the scripts for cancer, chemotherapy, chronic fatigue, general illness, and stress.

BREAST CANCER SCRIPT

THE TEAM
Intention: To eliminate breast cancer.

Find a comfortable place where you won't be disturbed, and sit in a comfortable chair. Now sit back and relax with both feet on the floor, and place your hands on the armrests of the chair or in your lap — whichever is comfortable for you.

Concentrate as you breathe deeply, letting the air come into your nose and out your mouth. Concentrate and breathe IN with the nose and OUT with the mouth. IN with the nose and OUT with the mouth. And IN with the nose and OUT with the mouth. Now let's concentrate on breathing OUT with the mouth and IN with the nose. And OUT with the mouth and IN with the nose. And OUT with the mouth and IN with the mouth.

Imagine you are in the most beautiful room you have ever seen. The carpet is your favorite color. The furniture is so beautiful. Look to your left and see a beautiful picture window. As you look out the window, you see a wonderful breathtaking view. In front of the window is a chair. Sit down in the chair and look out at the view. The chair is soft and comfortable. The view is so peaceful and you become very, very relaxed.

(Close your eyes for a moment and look at the view.)

As you are sitting looking out the window, you see the window change into a big TV screen. The view becomes fuzzy until you see that you are looking inside your breast. Look at the healthy tissue and the cancerous tissue. From the right of the screen, watch a line of very small dump trucks drive onto the screen. Watch the dump trucks park near the cancerous tissue. Now watch as crews of very tiny people come out of the dump trucks and stand before the cancerous tissue. Look and see how some of the tiny people have golden tools in their hands. Some of the tiny people have golden shovels and golden bags.

(Close your eyes for a moment and see these tiny people.)

Watch as the tiny people with the golden tools attack and dismantle the cancerous tissue. Watch the tiny people with the golden shovels and bags shovel up the bad tissue and place it in their golden bags. When each bag is full, watch the tiny people load the golden bags onto the dump trucks. Watch all the tiny people working as a team.

(Close your eyes for a moment and see the tiny people.)

Now watch as some of the tiny people have golden wands in their hands. These wands send out wonderful healing light. Wherever they point the wand a golden light comes out of the wand, healing the area it hits. Stopping the growth of bad cells. Continue to watch as the team gets rid of the bad tissue, packs it into bags, places the bags onto the dump trucks, and heals each area with golden light.

(Close your eyes for a moment and feel your body healing.)

When the trucks are full, watch as the team of tiny people get into the trucks and drive away, taking with them all the bad tissue, away from your body. You know you are healing. You feel the energy flowing through your body and are happy and peaceful. As the last truck drives off the screen and away from your body, you see the screen shift back to the beautiful picture window. You know you have healed today. This is your special place and you can come here whenever you need to.

You feel so healthy, relaxed, and joyful. These feelings will stay with you.

CHAPTER 12

Cancer and Chemotherapy

Cancer belongs to a large class of diseases known as neoplasms. Neoplasms, or tumors, are new tissue growth which does not follow the regular rules of metabolism and growth of normal cells in the body, and serves no function. Neoplastic cells can be classified as benign or malignant. Most malignant tumors have abnormalities in their DNA molecules. Cancer always denotes a malignant neoplasm. Cancers fall into four categories: 1) leukemias, which involve the blood-forming tissue; 2) sarcomas, which affect muscle, bone, cartilage, and connective tissue; 3) carcinomas, which affect skin, organs, mucous membranes, and glands; and 4) lymphomas, which affect the lymphatic system.

A carcinogen is a cancer-causing agent. Carcinogens can be chemical, biological, or physical. Here are some carcinogens: smoke, plant mold, some metals, prescribed hormones (e.g., estrogen replacement therapy); parasites; certain kinds of viruses; and ultraviolet and high-energy radiation. Usually cancer develops over an extended period of time after the initial exposure to a carcinogen. Cell aging, diet, heredity, poor nutrition, environmental factors, and hormone imbalances can help promote cancer.

Once a tumor progresses from benign to malignant, the cells develop additional abnormalities and start to grow more rapidly. The cells then start to metastasize, or spread, either through the bloodstream or lymphatic system to other parts of the body. Sometimes cancer can stop and remain dormant for years before continuing to grow.

Early diagnosis is advantageous in the treatment of cancer. Prevention through proper diet, nutrition, and exercise, elimination of potential environmental risk factors, and stress reduction can reduce the risk of cancer.

Traditional therapies include surgery, radiation, chemotherapy, and drug therapy. Most of these techniques destroy or weaken the body's natural immune system. Chemotherapy is systemic treatment of cancer using harmful, poisonous chemicals placed inside the body to destroy the cancer cells. Chemotherapy is effective in only a few types of cancers. However, for the majority of cancers, using chemotherapy to obtain a complete cure is uncommon. Chemotherapy is commonly used to extend a person's life. Many doctors will not use chemotherapy for themselves or their families.

The side effects of chemotherapy are many and vary with the type and amount of the toxic chemical received. The body is weakened because your immune system has to fight off the toxic chemical and its side effects in addition to the cancer. Before you make a choice to use chemotherapy, get all the facts. Research, ask questions, and demand answers about all the side effects of the drug.

If chemotherapy is your choice, you must truly feel and believe, beyond a doubt, that this method will work for you. In addition, you must build up and maintain your immune system at its peak performance before, during, and after each chemotherapy session to help your body minimize the debilitating side effects. Diet, supplements, and exercise become even more important if chemotherapy is your choice for healing cancer.

Natural therapies deal with cancer by using nontoxic biological substances (e.g., amino acid derivatives, shark cartilage); detoxification therapies (e.g., oxygen therapy, ozone therapy, colon cleansing); nutritional therapies (diet and supplements); herbal therapies; and mind-body therapies (e.g., hypnosis, visualization, biofeedback). Most of these techniques have few, if any, side effects. Natural therapies works on the whole person, boosting the immune system and changing the lifestyle to a healthier one. There are many different kinds of natural therapies that have been effective in the treatment for cancer. Work with antineoplastons, compounds found in the human blood and urine that fight abnormal cancer cells by reprogramming the cancer cells, has shown great promise in the fight against cancer. This therapy is a form of natural chemotherapy. Blood protein therapy is also another alternative therapy. Before making a decision as to which therapy is right for you, it is imperative that you do thorough research.

Cancer Relief Remedies

MENTAL ATTITUDE

Cause: hatred of some part of the self.

Cure: forgive and love yourself.

FOODS & DIET

Avoid: meat, processed food, animal and vegetable oils, white flour, sugar, salt, alcohol, caffeine, drugs, nicotine, artificial flavorings, colors, preservatives, peanuts, saturated fats; limit dairy foods.

Good Foods: low-fat, high-fiber, mostly vegetarian diet; whole grains, including brown rice, corn, alfalfa, wild rice; fruits and vegetables, including cauliflower, broccoli, kale, brussels sprouts, onions, spinach, cabbage, red and green peppers, turnips, strawberries, horseradish, radishes, eggplant, sweet potatoes, beets, tomatoes, avocados; yogurt; maitake and shiitake mushrooms; salt water fish; almonds, cashews, filberts, soybeans; kelp; flaxseed oil.

VITAMINS & SUPPLEMENTS

Multivitamin and mineral supplement with whole foods and enzymes, Vitamin C, A, E, B12, B6, beta carotene, bioflavonoids, germanium, SOD (superoxide desmutase), selenium, shark cartilage, DMG (dimethyl glycine), betaine hydrochloric acid, acidophilus, coenzyme Q10, and grape seed extract.

HERBS

Cumin, garlic, red clover, Essiac tea, green tea, cat's claw, pau d'arco, echinacea, aloe vera, dandelion.

AROMATHERAPY

Eucalyptus, hyssop, cypress, cedarwood..

The following scripts should be used in the morning and at night for at least six weeks. To optimize results, you may even want to try the scripts for breast cancer, chronic fatigue, general illness, and stress.

CANCER SCRIPTS

THE MIRROR IN THE SKY
Intention: To heal from cancer.

Find a comfortable place where you won't be disturbed, and sit in a comfortable chair. Now sit back and relax with both feet on the floor, and place your hands on the armrests of the chair or in your lap — whichever is comfortable for you.

Concentrate as you breathe deeply, letting the air come into your nose and out your mouth. Concentrate and breathe IN with the nose and OUT with the mouth. IN with the nose and OUT with the mouth. And IN with the nose and OUT with the mouth. Now let's concentrate on breathing OUT with the mouth and IN with the nose. And OUT with the mouth and IN with the nose. And OUT with the mouth and IN with the mouth.

Imagine yourself floating on a cloud in the sky. You are weightless and the cloud is so soft and supportive. Look around you and see the beautiful blue sky. It has different shades of blue; how beautiful it is! Look and feel the softness of the clouds around you. You are so very, very relaxed just floating on this cloud in the sky.

(Close your eyes for a moment and feel how relaxed you are.)

Stand up in the cloud and look to your left. The cloud has formed a path you can walk on. Start walking down the path. Feel how sturdy the clouds are beneath your feet. As you walk, watch as the mist from the clouds billows up around your ankles. It seems to make patterns and then disappear back into the clouds as you pass by. Look at the end of the path; there is a full-length mirror there. Walk to the mirror and stand before it. Gaze at your reflection in the mirror. You can see the outside and inside of your body. Now watch as your image in the mirror is surrounded by a beautiful white light. It is as if you have a halo of light surrounding your body from head to toe. Your image is completely surrounded by this white light.

(Close your eyes for a moment and see the white light.)

This white light feels soothing, yet filled with wonderful energy. Watch as the white light gets brighter and brighter. Now watch as this white light surrounding your body starts to enter inside your body.

Watch as this white light goes to any area that is diseased and illuminates it. Every area that is not working correctly and properly for you is being lit up with this healing white light. When each trouble spot in your body is covered with white light, feel the white light absorbing all the trouble. Drawing out any contamination, anything that is keeping you from being whole and healthy in this time, in this place, right now.

Watch and feel all the trouble spots being absorbed away from your body and into the white light.

(Close your eyes for a moment and feel the healing taking place.)

As each trouble spot is absorbed within the white light and away from your body, you feel this white healing light softly soothe each trouble spot and fill in each spot with healing light.

Watch and feel how the white light goes through your body cleansing, repairing, healing all the damaged areas of your body.

(Close your eyes for a moment and feel your body healing.)

Now breathe in very deeply and as you exhale slowly through the mouth, watch as the white light comes out of your body. With each exhalation, the white light is expelling the contamination out and away from your body. Take some time now and look at each trouble spot, and exhale it slowly and evenly out and away from the body. Feel the healing taking place. Feel the white light reconstructing the damaged cells, making you whole and perfect now.

(Close your eyes for a moment and see this happening.)

Now look at your image in the mirror. See how your body has healed. Look at your face. You feel happiness and joy because you know you are healing. Look in the mirror and see how healthy your body is. Feel the energy and power of your body. Turn away from the mirror and walk down the cloud path. Lie down in the clouds. You are weightless and floating. You feel happy, healthy, and relaxed. These feelings will stay with you.

CHEMOTHERAPY SCRIPTS

THE KNIGHT*

*To be used prior to chemotherapy.
Intention: To build up the immune system.

Find a comfortable place where you won't be disturbed, and sit in a comfortable chair. Now sit back and relax with both feet on the floor, and place your hands on the armrests of the chair or in your lap — whichever is comfortable for you.

Concentrate as you breathe deeply, letting the air come into your nose and out your mouth. Concentrate and breathe IN with the nose and OUT with the mouth. IN with the nose and OUT with the mouth. And IN with the nose and OUT with the mouth. Now let's concentrate on breathing OUT with the mouth and IN with the nose. And OUT with the mouth and IN with the nose. And OUT with the mouth and IN with the mouth.

Imagine yourself in a wide open field. The grass is green. The sky is blue with gently floating clouds. The air temperature is exactly right for you. The sun is shining and warm on your body. The field is surrounded by a forest of tall trees. The trees are tall and gently swaying in the breeze. Sit down on the soft, lush grass. It is quiet and peaceful. Reach up your hand with the palm facing up and raise it to the sky. Watch as a ray of golden sunshine comes out of the sun and goes to the palm of your hand. Now watch as the golden ray of sun that is in the palm of your hand begins to take on a shape. As you watch you see a tiny medieval knight on a white horse. Watch as he takes shape. See his armor glinting in the sun. Look at his face. He is kind, yet strong. Feel the power coming from this tiny medieval knight. Look at his left hand. He is holding a golden sword. Look at his right hand. He is holding a golden wand. Now watch as the knight rides into your body. Watch him as he rides to your spleen. Watch as the good lymphocytes come out to follow him. Now watch as the golden wand sends out a golden light. Watch as this golden light surrounds each lymphocyte, giving each one extra power, extra strength. Now watch as he rides through your body, using his sword to cut down all the bad cells. Tossing each bad cell to the lymphocytes, which finish destroying and killing each bad cell.

(Close your eyes for a moment and watch the knight and the lymphocytes.)

Now watch as the knight rides to your thymus gland. See the T4 cells come out to greet him. See the golden light of his wand surround each one. They now have extra power and strength. Watch as his sword cuts down the bad cells. See how the T4 cells fight and destroy your illness. See and hear the knight go through your body calling to your T8 white blood cells. These cells are his allies that will help to fight your illness. Watch as the knight finds a trouble spot and fights it with his allies.

(Close your eyes for a moment and watch the knight and his allies.)

When the knight is done, watch the knight ride back to the palm of your hand the same way he went in.

Stand up in the field with your palm extended, holding the knight and his horse in its center. Look at the knight and see him salute you. Thank him for helping you and then gently close your hand and place the knight in your pocket. You know he is your own special knight who will protect you whenever you need him. Whenever you call on him he will be there. Look around you and see the trees, the sky, the sun. You are peaceful because you know you are winning your health. You are happy that you are healing. These feelings will stay with you.

THE HEALING KNIGHT*

To be used during chemotherapy.
Intention: To aid healing.

Relax and get comfortable. There is no fear, just a sense of deep, deep relaxation.

Concentrate as you breathe deeply, letting the air come into your nose and out your mouth. Concentrate and breathe IN with the nose and OUT with the mouth. IN with the nose and OUT with the mouth. And IN with the nose and OUT with the mouth. Now let's concentrate on breathing OUT with the mouth and IN with the nose. And OUT with the mouth and IN with the nose. And OUT with the mouth and IN with the mouth.

Imagine your special tiny knight on his white horse in the palm of your hand. Look at his beautiful horse, his shining armor, his face. He is smiling at you. You feel his strength and power. You know that he will be helping you. In his hands he has his golden wand. Watch as he points his golden wand towards your body where the chemicals are going in. Watch him ride into your body, following the same path as the chemicals. As he rides through your body and points the golden wand, a golden light comes out of it. The light is healing and comforting and surrounds each good cell, protecting each one from harm from the chemicals. Now see the chemicals destroying the bad cells. Feel the golden light hit the good cells, protecting them from the chemicals, each and every one. Feel the golden light follow the chemicals. Protecting, soothing, healing each area.

Watch as the cancer is being destroyed. Feel the light protecting you. You are happy and strong knowing you are healing from within. You will keep this feeling with you.

THE HEALING WATERFALL*

To be used after chemotherapy
Intention: To eliminate cancer.

Find a comfortable place where you won't be disturbed, and sit in a comfortable chair. Now sit back and relax with both feet on the floor, and place your hands on the armrests of the chair or in your lap — whichever is comfortable for you.

Concentrate as you breathe deeply, letting the air come into your nose and out your mouth. Concentrate and breathe IN with the nose and OUT with the mouth. IN with the nose and OUT with the mouth. And IN with the nose and OUT with the mouth. Now let's concentrate on breathing OUT with the mouth and IN with the nose. And OUT with the mouth and IN with the nose. And OUT with the mouth and IN with the mouth.

Imagine yourself in a green, grassy meadow. There is a pond with a beautiful waterfall nearby. See the flowers and the stones. Look at the colors around you. Hear the birds singing in the trees, singing sweet melodies among the quiet. The air smells fresh and sweet. It is so peaceful and relaxing here.

(Close your eyes for a moment and feel the peacefulness.)

Look at the waterfall. Hear the water trickling down over the rocks. See the water gently flowing down, forming a shallow pool at the base of the waterfall. See how the water sparkles in the sun. It is so peaceful and calm here and you know that this waterfall can heal you. This is your private place. You are alone and no one can enter here. Take off your clothes and lay them down on a large dry rock. Step into the pool. The water temperature is just right for you. Feel how the water is cleansing and healing your body as you step deeper and deeper in the pool.

(Close your eyes for a moment and feel the healing water.)

Walk over to the waterfall and step under it. Feel the healing water cleansing and healing your body. The healing is stronger here, and you feel the energy course through your body as the water hits it. Now watch as the water turns into many colored rainbow lights. They are glinting and bright. How beautiful this is. Feel the rainbow lights as they touch you. They may be red, yellow, green, blue, silver, gold — any and all colors. The lights are soothing, healing, magical. Feel how the lights go into your body, making you feel cleansed, whole, healed. Making you strong. Making you perfect and whole now.

(Close your eyes for a moment and feel the healing taking place.)

When you are ready, step out from under the waterfall. Watch as the rainbow lights turn back into the gently flowing water. Wade across the pool of healing water. As you step on the land, you are completely dry.

Put your clothes on. You feel strong, healthy and at peace. You feel relaxed, peaceful, yet filled with energy. These feelings will stay with you.

CHAPTER 13

Cataracts

The eyeball is about an inch in diameter. This ball is covered in the back by a coating called the sclera, also known as the white of the eye. In the front of the eye is a transparent tissue called the cornea. Under the sclera is the choroid, a membrane that contains the blood vessels that nourish the eye. The iris or pigmented diaphragm of the eye and its central pupil are located behind the center of the cornea. Behind the iris is the transparent lens.

A cataract is the loss of transparency of the lens. The lens becomes cloudy or opaque, thickens, and has difficulty in focusing and admitting light. (This is different than small lens opacities, which are common and may be present from birth.) Cataracts can arise from congenital sources or as the result of trauma, heavy metal poisoning, diabetes, radiation exposure, and steroids. However, the main cause of cataracts is aging; these are called senile cataracts. Senile cataracts occur gradually over a period of time and normally are painless. They usually affect people over age 65 and are often caused by free radical damage in the body. Your body releases free radicals when certain fats are broken down and when there is exposure to ultra-violet light, low-level radiation (e.g., X-rays), or chemical pollutants. The free radicals are reactive chemical fragments that attach to the eye proteins, cell membranes, and enzymes. This is what causes cataracts. Avoiding fluorinated and chlorinated water aids in cataract prevention, as does drinking filtered water. Limit dairy products and heated saturated fats and oils, because they promote lens damage and the formation of free radicals.

Cataract Relief Remedies

MENTAL ATTITUDE
Cause: not wanting to see the future.
Cure: create a plan and take action.

FOODS & DIET
Avoid: heated fats, saturated fats, animal fats, oils, sugar, dairy products, and antihistamines.
Good Foods: Pure water; carrots; squash; sweet potatoes; green veg-

etables, including broccoli, watercress, parsley, spinach; rose hips; cherries; blueberries; grapefruit; royal jelly; alfalfa; lentils; molasses; tuna; salmon; sardines.

VITAMINS & SUPPLEMENTS
Multivitamin and mineral supplement with whole foods and enzymes, Vitamin C, A, E, B2, B6, B complex, L-lysine, selenium, zinc, riboflavin, manganese, beta carotene, bioflavonoids.

HERBS
Cumin, garlic, aloe vera, bilberry.

AROMATHERAPY
Lavender, myrrh, frankincense, sandalwood.

The following scripts should be used in the morning and at night for at least six weeks. To optimize results, you may even want to try the scripts for general illness.

CATARACT SCRIPTS

THE TROPICAL ISLAND
Intention: To eliminate cataracts.

Find a comfortable place where you won't be disturbed, and sit in a comfortable chair. Now sit back and relax with both feet on the floor, and place your hands on the armrests of the chair or in your lap — whichever is comfortable for you.

Concentrate as you breathe deeply, letting the air come into your nose and out your mouth. Concentrate and breathe IN with the nose and OUT with the mouth. IN with the nose and OUT with the mouth. And IN with the nose and OUT with the mouth. Now let's concentrate on breathing OUT with the mouth and IN with the nose. And OUT with the mouth and IN with the nose. And OUT with the mouth and IN with the mouth.

Imagine you are on a tropical island. The ocean is the most beautiful blues and greens. The palm trees are gently swaying in the tropical breeze. The smell of exotic spices and lavender fill the air. The sky is blue with just some soft, wispy clouds floating by. You are standing by the ocean and feel so relaxed as the tropical breezes gently float across your body. You are wearing a bathing suit in exotic colors and are an excellent swimmer and scuba diver. You know that the waters are safe and nothing can harm you. Look down to your left; you see a mask and all the right equipment that you need. Look out over the water and see a beautiful reef close by. Put on the equipment and begin to swim towards the reef. You swim slowly and are very relaxed without a care or worry in the world.

(Close your eyes for a moment and feel how relaxed you are.)

When you get to the reef, dive down. It is not too deep. Through your mask you see the beautiful fish just swimming by. Look at the beautiful plants and watch the colors on the bottom of the ocean floor. How very serene and beautiful this is. You feel free, happy, and safe. Just observing and watching all the sea life.

(Close your eyes for a moment and see all the beauty.)

Look to your right; there is a cave that is not too far away. Swim over and enter the cave. In the cave you see an old pirate chest buried in the sand. Swim over to the pirate chest and start clearing away the sand until the whole chest is exposed. The water around you starts to become very cloudy and there is a film on your mask that you can hardly see through. Your mask is becoming more and more cloudy. You try to clear the outside of the mask but it only gets cloudier. You are not afraid because you know you are in control. You can dimly see the chest; go over and open it. The chest is filled with gold coins. These coins start to radiate a golden light. This golden light pierces the film on the mask and starts breaking it away. Watch as the water and the golden light remove all the cloudiness from your mask. Bit by bit by bit. Slowly making your vision clearer and clearer. Feel the golden light clearing your mask in exactly the right way for you.

(Close your eyes for a moment and feel the mask becoming clear.)

Watch until all the film is gone and you can see clearly. See the golden light of the coins shining brightly. You feel so wonderful as you look at all the beautiful things around you. Take a handful of the golden coins and put them in a pouch at your waist. Swim out of the cave and back to the beach. Get out of the water and sit in the sand looking through your mask. You can see clearly, all the film is gone.

Take the golden coins out of your pouch and look at them. They are magic coins and they glint gently in the sunlight. You smile, knowing you have done great work today. You feel happy and relaxed and you will keep this feeling with you.

THE CLEANER
Intention: To eliminate cataracts.

Find a comfortable place where you won't be disturbed, and sit in a comfortable chair. Now sit back and relax with both feet on the floor, and place your hands on the armrests of the chair or in your lap — whichever is comfortable for you.

Concentrate as you breathe deeply, letting the air come into your nose and out your mouth. Concentrate and breathe IN with the nose and OUT with the mouth. IN with the nose and OUT with the mouth. And IN with the nose and OUT with the mouth. Now let's concentrate on breathing OUT with the mouth and IN with the nose. And OUT with the mouth and IN with the nose. And OUT with the mouth and IN with the mouth.

Imagine you are a very tiny cleaner. You have all the tools you need. Look around you and see that you are inside your eye. You are actually in back of the lens of your eye and you can see a milky film over the lens. It looks opaque and you can't seem to see through the lens and out to the outside world.

(Close your eyes for a moment and look at your lens.)

You are very relaxed because you are a very good cleaner and have all the right tools to get the job done. Look to your left and pick up a spray bottle filled with rainbow colored liquid and a special polishing cloth. You know that this bottle contains a healing spray that can dissolve the film on the lens and the polishing cloth can wipe away any residue that is left. Proceed to start cleaning and polishing the film away. Ever so gently, methodically spray the healing liquid and polish with the polishing cloth, cleaning the lens. Keep cleaning and polishing until your lens becomes clear.

(Close your eyes for a moment and see how you are cleaning and polishing.)

When you are done, look into the lens; you can now see the outside world very clearly. Step back and smile; you are so happy and this feeling will stay with you.

CHAPTER 14

Chronic Fatigue Syndrome and Epstein-Barr Virus

Chronic fatigue syndrome and Epstein-Barr virus (EBV) are controversial diseases. Some United States medical establishments still deny these diseases even exist. In Europe and other parts of the world they are recognized diseases. Often these diseases are misdiagnosed as psychosomatic illness, hypochondria, or depression because routine medical tests do not show that a medical problem exists. Explanations for the cause of these diseases have ranged from airborne virus to bacteria found in meat to environmental factors. Viral causes that have been implicated in contributing to the chronic fatigue syndrome include but are not limited to: herpes, Epstein-Barr, adenovirus, enterovirus, and coxsackievirus. EBV is a herpes virus that also causes mononucleosis. High levels of EBV antibodies are found in the blood with Epstein-Barr virus infection. Fibromyalgia (a muscle disorder) and *Candida albicans* (a fungus infection) have been found in many people with chronic fatigue syndrome and Epstein-Barr virus. Today no one is really sure what causes chronic fatigue syndrome or Epstein-Barr.

These diseases are so hard to diagnose because the symptoms vary with each individual and seem to hit people in their weakest spots. Five major categories of symptoms have been identified and related to chronic fatigue syndrome and Epstein-Barr: an immune system breakdown with low adrenal function; thyroid imbalances; hypoglycemia; Vitamin B deficiencies; and cerebral allergies. The symptoms can include any or all of the following: viral infection, headaches, flulike symptoms, joint pain, vision changes, sensitivity to light and heat, swollen glands, ear balance problems, sore throat, sleep disturbances, intestinal problems, loss of appetite, memory and concentration problems, distorted sentences, depression, anxiety, panic attacks, and debilitating fatigue.

Traditional medicine, if it even recognizes the diseases, provides drug therapies to fight individual symptoms. Natural therapies include vitamin therapies, herbal therapies, dietary and lifestyle changes, homeopathy, acupuncture, visualization, self-hypnosis, exercise, and stress-reducing techniques. A combination of a dietary changes, vitamins, supplements, herbs, and self-hypnosis worked for me.

Chronic Fatigue and EBV Relief Remedies

MENTAL ATTITUDE

Cause: fear or inability to change, or a false desire for self-importance.
Cure: take action and be forgiving and love oneself.

FOODS & DIET

Avoid: wheat, white flour, white rice, all grains (except rye, corn, quinoa), cheese and dairy products (except eggs, butter, yogurt), meat (except lamb, chicken, turkey, venison, rabbit, duck), fermentation products, alcohol, vinegar, sugar, salt, carbonated drinks, coffee, caffeine, food colorings, preservatives, and additives, processed foods, citrus and all other fruits (except tropical fruits), orange roughy, trout, oils (except flaxseed, borage), peanuts, macadamia nuts, yeast, iceberg lettuce, tomatoes, potatoes.

Good Foods: rye, corn, quinoa, oat bran, brown rice, wild rice, goat cheese, eggs, butter, yogurt, lamb, chicken, turkey, venison, duck, olive oil, safflower oil, evening primrose oil, sweet potatoes, yams, bananas, kiwi, pineapple, almonds, fish, guava, papaya, avocados, pecans, walnuts, cashews, vegetables, royal jelly, spirulina, blue-green algae, herbal teas.

VITAMINS & SUPPLEMENTS

Multivitamin and mineral supplement with whole foods and enzymes, Vitamin C, A, E, B6, B complex, calcium, magnesium, beta carotene, bioflavonoids, manganese, quercetin, pycnogenol, zinc, coenzyme Q10, selenium, chromium picolinate, lecithin, amino acid complex, acidophilus.

HERBS

Pau d'arco, grape seed extract, green tea, oregano, cumin, coriander, basil, astragalus, ginkgo biloba, burdock root, red clover, garlic.

AROMATHERAPY

Lavender, neroli, rose, benzoin.

The following scripts should be used in the morning and at night for at least six weeks. To optimize results, you may even want to try the scripts for general illness, anxiety, allergy, depression, lack of energy, headaches, insomnia, memory loss, pain, vertigo, and stress.

CHRONIC FATIGUE/EBV SCRIPTS

THE TENNIS GAME
Intention: To eliminate the disease.

Find a comfortable place where you won't be disturbed, and sit in a comfortable chair. Now sit back and relax with both feet on the floor, and place your hands on the armrests of the chair or in your lap — whichever is comfortable for you.

Concentrate as you breathe deeply, letting the air come into your nose and out your mouth. Concentrate and breathe IN with the nose and OUT with the mouth. IN with the nose and OUT with the mouth. And IN with the nose and OUT with the mouth. Now let's concentrate on breathing OUT with the mouth and IN with the nose. And OUT with the mouth and IN with the nose. And OUT with the mouth and IN with the mouth.

Imagine that you are on a tennis court and you are playing a piano. There is a tennis racquet very close to you. The music that you are playing on the piano is very sweet and enticing. You are an excellent piano player and the melodies are haunting and beautiful. Look to your right and see the net of the tennis court. See how the sun sparkles on the net. Look past the net and on the other side you see a big box. As you continue playing your beautiful music, you see a virus jump out of the box. It was drawn out of the box by your beautiful music. Stand up and pick up your tennis racquet. Watch as the virus flies through the air, coming over the net towards you. Swing the tennis racquet and hit the virus away from you. Watch as the virus hits the racquet, how it is tossed away from your body and disappears. Watch as other viruses come out of the box one by one. Feel the tremendous power and agility coming through your body. As you swing your racquet, it hits each virus away from your body and you watch each one disappear. You cannot miss because you are strong and powerful. Watch each virus come out of the box and swing your racquet and hit them away from your body. Watch as each one disappears.

(Close your eyes for a moment and see yourself hitting each virus.)

Whenever the viruses stop coming out of the box, sit back down at your piano and play the enticing music. Watch as more viruses come out of the box. Watch as you swing your tennis racquet, hit them, and see them disappear. You are happy because you know you are healing. You feel powerful because you know you are winning the game. Continue to hit them as long as you want. When you are done you feel happy and healthy, and this feeling will stay with you.

THE MAGIC FLOWER
Intention: To eliminate the disease.

Find a comfortable place where you won't be disturbed, and sit in a comfortable chair. Now sit back and relax with both feet on the floor, and place your hands on the armrests of the chair or in your lap — whichever is comfortable for you.

Concentrate as you breathe deeply, letting the air come into your nose and out your mouth. Concentrate and breathe IN with the nose and OUT with the mouth. IN with the nose and OUT with the mouth. And IN with the nose and OUT with the mouth. Now let's concentrate on breathing OUT with the mouth and IN with the nose. And OUT with the mouth and IN with the nose. And OUT with the mouth and IN with the mouth.

Imagine you are walking on a path in the woods. Look at the trees around you. You are feeling very relaxed and happy. The trees have spots of sunlight reflecting through their branches. As the sunlight lands on the path, it sparkles. As you walk down the path, the sparkling light looks so beautiful in its ever-changing patterns. As you turn to the left of the path, you see a stream. There is big flat wide rock there and you sit on the rock. As you sit so quietly and relaxed, listen to the birds singing in the trees. Hear the stream babbling softly. As you sit on the rock, you notice the most beautiful flower you have ever seen. It is different and has multi-colored petals. It seems to sparkle and shine as the sun hits it. Pick the flower and bring it close to your nose and smell it. It has a sweet scent that seems to be very, very healing. As you breathe in the scent of the flower, you feel an energy come in through your nose and enter your body.

(Close your eyes for a moment and feel this energy.)

This energy makes you calm and centered. Your eyes become very focused and clear. All the physical stress in your body seems to relax as you smell the scent of this wonderful flower. You are so calm and your body feels very balanced.

As you breathe deeply into the flower, you know that the scent is healing your body. The aches and pains just disappear. Feel the flower's energy go through your body. Healing your symptoms one by one. Feel the flower giving you energy. Healing you right now.

(Close your eyes for a moment and feel the healing taking place.)

Focus on smelling the flower and feel its energy take away your joint pain, curing all the aches in your body, making you strong and healthy. Continue to breathe this wonderful flower until you feel a shift in the energy of your body. You feel this gentle warm energy go into your head, down your back, to the bottom of your feet. Feel this energy travel up the front of your legs, your abdomen, your chest, and all the way to the top of your head. Feel the healing taking place throughout your body as this energy passes over each trouble spot.

(Close your eyes for a moment and feel this healing energy.)

You feel energized and awake with exactly the right energy for you. What a wonderful flower this is. Such a wonderful gift. Take the flower and put it in your pocket. The magic flower will always be fresh and a source of energy for you whenever you need it.

You feel happy, pain-free, balanced, and filled with energy, and this feeling will stay with you.

CHAPTER 15

Colds and Flu

The common cold is an infection of the upper respiratory tract, including infection of the mucus membranes of the nose (rhinitis). It can be caused by one or more of two hundred known viruses. Cold viruses are spread by air, or by direct contact with someone who is infected. Some of the symptoms of the common cold include: watery eyes, sneezing, fever, sore throat, muscle aches, headaches, head congestion, and coughing.

Influenza or flu symptoms are caused by a virus. The symptoms are like those of a cold but may also include: chills, weakness, nausea, high fever, and dry throat or dry cough. The flu is an infectious disease of the respiratory tract. Flus can be seasonal and occur most frequently from late December through mid-March. Flus make people more susceptible to sinus and ear problems, bronchitis, and pneumonia.

The flu usually lasts from 3 to 7 days. A period of weakness and depression usually follows. Bed rest and fluids are the best treatment. Sometimes antibiotics are given to prevent pneumonia. Antibiotics do not affect the flu virus itself, and they are ineffectual in destroying it. Flu viruses are constantly changing, which makes flu vaccines only partly successful. Vaccines can produce debilitating side effects. Children with flu infection should avoid aspirin, because taking aspirin during a viral illness has been linked to Reye's syndrome, a disorder that can result in coma or death.

Keeping the immune system strong and healthy is the best way to fight colds and flu. Proper diet, vitamin and nutritional supplements, adequate rest, exercise, and stress reduction boost the immune system to work at peak performance.

Americans spend more than a billion dollars a year on nonprescription cold remedies. Decongestants relieve swelling and congestion of the nasal passages and have side effects of fatigue, nervousness and insomnia. Analgesics relieve fever, aches and pain, but sometimes a low-grade fever is beneficial to fight off infection. Cough medicines may be expectorants or antitussives. Expectorants increase the amount of phlegm and decrease phlegm's thickness. Antitussives reduce cough frequency, but remember that coughing is the body's way to clear the lungs. Antihistamines decrease the swelling of small blood vessels in the nose, which helps reduce sneezing, but antihistamines have the side effect of drowsiness. Some combinations of over-the-counter cold remedies may work against each other, so be careful of what you take so that it is not counterproductive to the result you want.

When you get a cold, it is best to remain active to loosen up mucus and fluids in the body. With flu, liquids and bed rest are recommended. Natural methods to fight colds and flu include: herbal therapy (e.g., echinacea, goldenseal), vitamin therapy (e.g., zinc, Vitamin C), homeopathy, and aromatherapy.

Cold and Flu Relief Remedies

MENTAL ATTITUDE
Cause: indecision.
Cure: make decisions that produce action.

FOODS & DIET
Avoid: dairy products, alcohol, caffeine, food colorings, preservatives, and additives, processed foods.
Good Foods: citrus fruit, chicken, turkey, cabbage, red and green peppers, horseradish, cantaloupe, radishes, elderberries, papaya, olive oil, walnuts.

VITAMINS & SUPPLEMENTS
Multivitamin and mineral supplement with whole foods and enzymes, Vitamin C, A, B complex, garlic, L-lysine, zinc, acidophilus.

HERBS
Pau d'arco, basil, garlic, ginger, echinacea, goldenseal, catnip, boneset, lemon balm.

AROMATHERAPY
Oregano, basil, black pepper, eucalyptus, peppermint, rosemary, cypress.

The following scripts should be used in the morning and at night. To optimize results, you may even want to try the scripts for general illness, allergy, asthma/breathing, lack of energy, and headache.

COLD AND FLU SCRIPTS

CHICKEN SOUP
Intention: To eliminate cold and flu symptoms.

Find a comfortable place where you won't be disturbed, and sit in a comfortable chair. Now sit back and relax with both feet on the floor, and place your hands on the armrests of the chair or in your lap — whichever is comfortable for you.

Concentrate as you breathe deeply, letting the air come into your nose and out your mouth. Concentrate and breathe IN with the nose and OUT with the mouth. IN with the nose and OUT with the mouth. And IN with the nose and OUT with the mouth. Now let's concentrate on breathing OUT with the mouth and IN with the nose. And OUT with the mouth and IN with the nose. And OUT with the mouth and IN with the mouth.

Imagine that you are in a kitchen. It is so modern and has every convenience possible. Look over to your right and see a big, modern stove. As you walk over to the stove you see a covered pot on the stove. Take off the cover of the pot. It smells so good. There is a rich, warm, golden soup broth in the pot that is bubbling gently. The pot seems to be filled with energy. You start to crave some of the soup because you know that it will be the best soup you have ever tasted. Smell the aroma and feel the energy.

(Close your eyes for a moment and smell the soup.)

There are a ladle, a bowl, and a spoon on the counter near the stove. Pick up the ladle and put some of the golden soup into the bowl. Take the bowl and sit down at the kitchen table. As you sit down, you see a window that has the most beautiful view. Stop for a moment and look at this peaceful, calming view. Everything is crystal clear and you know that this is how you see your life. You feel that you know what to do in every situation. Feeling a surge of power going through you, look down at the soup.

(Close your eyes for a moment and feel the power.)

Pick up the spoon and start to eat the soup. You feel the soup's warmth as it goes down into your stomach. This warmth starts to radiate through your body. It goes into your throat and you feel your throat begin to heal.

(Close your eyes for a moment and feel your throat healing.)

Take another spoonful of soup and eat it. It is the best soup you have ever tasted. Now the warmth seems to spread into your respiratory tract, healing you, soothing you. Feel the warmth absorbing the virus and take it away from your body. Feel the warmth of the soup healing you. You are able to breathe easier. The warmth of the soup is helping you heal right now.

(Close your eyes for a moment and feel the healing.)

Take another spoonful of soup. Feel the warmth going into your nose and any other place in your body that needs healing. Feel the warmth of the soup healing you. Soothing your body. Eat as much soup as you need, and feel the warmth heal you. When you are done, you feel healthy, happy and rested. You have energy and purpose. You are calm and centered and feel so good. This feeling will stay with you.

THE DIAMOND
Intention: To eliminate cold and flu symptoms.

Find a comfortable place where you won't be disturbed, and sit in a comfortable chair. Now sit back and relax with both feet on the floor, and place your hands on the armrests of the chair or in your lap — whichever is comfortable for you.

Concentrate as you breathe deeply, letting the air come into your nose and out your mouth. Concentrate and breathe IN with the nose and OUT with the mouth. IN with the nose and OUT with the mouth. And IN with the nose and OUT with the mouth. Now let's concentrate on breathing OUT with the mouth and IN with the nose. And OUT with the mouth and IN with the nose. And OUT with the mouth and IN with the mouth.

Imagine you are in a cave. It is dark but at the back of the cave you see a light. Walk towards the light. When you get to the back of the cave you see a diamond embedded in the cave wall. The diamond is filled with white light and is lighting the back of the cave where you are standing.

Watch as the rays of white light come out of the diamond. You know that this is healing light. Stand in front of the diamond and feel the healing rays enter into your body.

(Close your eyes for a moment and feel the healing light.)

The white diamond light goes to each part of your body that has a symptom. Feel that symptom heal in the white diamond light. Healing you wherever you need healing. Whatever you need, the diamond light provides it for you. You feel, know, and trust this. Feel the healing of mind, body, and spirit that is being done right now, in this time, in this place.

(Close your eyes for a moment and feel the healing.)

Stand in the diamond light as long as you need to. When you are done, walk out of the cave. You feel healthy and whole. You feel filled with energy and this feeling will stay with you.

CHAPTER 16

Constipation

Constipation is the difficult or infrequent passage of feces out of the body. When feces are detained from leaving the body, water is absorbed from the feces, which then dry and harden, making them difficult to eliminate. When this happens, the waste material continually overloads the bowel muscles and they become weak and lose their tone, which can lead to chronic constipation. Harmful toxins and bacteria may then develop, and this can lead to body odor, gas, fatigue, diverticulitis, hiatus hernia, indigestion, bloating, insomnia, headaches, hemorrhoids, obesity, *Candida*, and thyroid disease.

Insufficient amounts of fiber and fluids in the diet, lack of exercise, muscle disorders, aging, structural abnormalities, antidepressants and pain-killer drugs, and bowel disease can cause constipation. In most cases, constipation is due to junk food and poor diet.

Excessive use of enemas and laxatives can lead to irregularity, hemorrhoids, and bowel irritation. Waste material should pass out of the body within 18 to 24 hours after eating, on a daily basis.

Increasing fiber and fluid in the diet, adjusting your diet to a healthy one, getting regular exercise, and using stress-reduction techniques can help constipation.

Constipation Relief Remedies

MENTAL ATTITUDE
Cause: holding on to the past.
Cure: live in the moment.

FOODS & DIET
Avoid: dairy products, alcohol, caffeine, sugar, salt, food colorings, preservatives, and additives, processed foods.
Good Foods: garlic, papaya, apple pectin, broccoli, tomatoes, sweet potatoes, oat bran, grapefruit, kiwi, wheat bran, yogurt, rice bran, wild rice, artichokes, strawberries.

VITAMINS & SUPPLEMENTS

Multivitamin and mineral supplement with whole foods and enzymes, Vitamin C, D, E, acidophilus, calcium, magnesium.

HERBS

Alfalfa, aloe vera, basil, cascara sagrada, flaxseed, garlic, milk thistle, psyllium.

AROMATHERAPY

Black pepper, camphor, marjoram, dill, fennel.

The following scripts should be used in the morning and at night for at least six weeks. To optimize results, you may even want to try the scripts for general illness.

CONSTIPATION SCRIPTS

THE GOLDEN WATER
Intention: To eliminate constipation.

Find a comfortable place where you won't be disturbed, and sit in a comfortable chair. Now sit back and relax with both feet on the floor, and place your hands on the armrests of the chair or in your lap — whichever is comfortable for you.

Concentrate as you breathe deeply, letting the air come into your nose and out your mouth. Concentrate and breathe IN with the nose and OUT with the mouth. IN with the nose and OUT with the mouth. And IN with the nose and OUT with the mouth. Now let's concentrate on breathing OUT with the mouth and IN with the nose. And OUT with the mouth and IN with the nose. And OUT with the mouth and IN with the mouth.

Imagine that you are in a garden. The sun is shining and the breeze is soft and gentle. It feels warm against your skin. You can smell the fresh-mown grass and all the flowers. The birds are singing gaily in the trees. It is such a lovely day. In the middle of the garden is a table. On the table is a clear glass pitcher of sparkling water. Look at the water and see that it contains tiny gold flecks. They sparkle and glimmer in the sun. The flecks in the water are very good for you. You feel and know this. In this garden it seems that you are fearless and courageous. You realize that life is a process of give and take, and you are in control of this process.

(Close your eyes for a moment and feel how fearless you are.)

You feel free in the garden and you trust that everything is really okay. You are filled with positive energy and you pick up the pitcher and pour yourself a glass of this special water. Drink the water. The water goes down your throat and into your digestive tract. Feel how the golden flecks in the water sparkle in your body. The flecks are healing you as it goes throughout your digestive tract. Now feel the golden-flecked water reach your intestines and colon. Soothing the sides of your colon, healing everything that needs to be healed.

(Close your eyes for a moment and feel the healing taking place.)

Feel the water absorbing into all your muscles, making them strong and giving them good tone. Feel this now. The golden-flecked water is throughout your digestive tract, making you able to process and absorb food correctly. Making you regular in elimination. Making everything in perfect working order. You know this is happening right now.

(Close your eyes for a moment and feel the healing.)

If you need more water, keep drinking as much as you need. After each drink, feel how the gold-flecked water is healing you. Giving you what you need. Empowering you to deal with your feelings and repairing your body at the same time. You know that everything inside and outside your body is perfect in every way. You desire to eat only the right foods for your body. You desire to drink the right amount of liquids for your body every day. Everything in your body is working correctly and properly. You feel balanced, centered, and happy. These feelings will stay with you.

THE BOX
Intention: To eliminate constipation.

Find a comfortable place where you won't be disturbed, and sit in a comfortable chair. Now sit back and relax with both feet on the floor, and place your hands on the armrests of the chair or in your lap — whichever is comfortable for you.

Concentrate as you breathe deeply, letting the air come into your nose and out your mouth. Concentrate and breathe IN with the nose and OUT with the mouth. IN with the nose and OUT with the mouth. And IN with the nose and OUT with the mouth. Now let's concentrate on breathing OUT with the mouth and IN with the nose. And OUT with the mouth and IN with the nose. And OUT with the mouth and IN with the mouth.

Imagine you are in a box. The box surrounds your body and it is very tight and close around you. There is hardly any room for you to move in this box. Take your hand and feel the insides of the box. It is hard and you feel so constricted and confined.

(Close your eyes for a moment and feel the box.)

Look up to the left-hand corner of the box; there is a hole there. Coming in from the hole is a bright white light. Look at the light and see how it seems to get brighter and brighter. You feel calm and peaceful in this white light. Feel how the light starts to surround your body inside the box. The air in the box seems to get lighter. Reach out a hand and touch the sides of the box. There seems to be more room inside now than there was before.

(Close your eyes for a moment and feel the box.)

Now you feel the white light circling your body, making you lighter as it extends the box away from your body. Look down at your feet; you see the bottom of the box is now covered with white light. You are able to move more freely in the box. The box has even more room than it did before.

Look back to the bottom of your feet and watch as the white light seems to disintegrate the bottom of the box, just making it melt away.

(Close your eyes for a moment and see the bottom of the box opening.)

The white light has given you superhuman strength. You feel this as you lift the box up and over your head and throw it behind you. You feel so peaceful as the white light lifts away from your body, leaving you whole and perfect right now. Feel the air flowing freely around you. You feel your body responding and you know that all of your body's systems are in good working order.

Feeling happy, healthy, and relaxed, you know this feeling will stay with you.

CHAPTER 17

Depression

Depression is an affective disorder that involves the body, mind, and spirit. There are many types of depression. Depression can be transient or last a lifetime. The symptoms of depression can include: poor appetite or overeating, weight loss or gain, insomnia or increased sleep, inability to concentrate, agitation, loss of interest, irritability, indecisiveness, feelings of worthlessness, guilt, self-reproach, fatigue, energy loss, headaches, backaches, digestive disorders, inability to perform sexually or decreased sexual drive, and recurrent thoughts of death or suicide.

Not all these symptoms occur in an individual who is depressed, but some or many are present.

For psychiatrists to treat depression, at least four of these symptoms must be experienced daily and be present for two weeks. In psychological terms, reactive depressions are associated with the loss of or separation from an object or a person. Endogenous depressions are associated with delusions and hallucinations. Unipolar depression consists of depressive episodes that may recur several times or more throughout a person's life. Bipolar depression, or manic depression, consists of alternate episodes of depression and mania.

Brain chemicals called neurotransmitters carry impulses between the nerve cells which regulate behavior. The way these neurotransmitters work is very intricate. The physical cause of depression is the depletion of these neurotransmitters (e.g., endorphin, norepinephrine, serotonin, dopamine) in specific brain areas. Serotonin eases tension, while norepinephrine and dopamine cause alertness. Depletion of neurotransmitters have many causes. Nutritional deficiencies may occur from excessive intake of alcohol, sugar, and caffeine. Depression can be triggered by stress, traumatic events, brain imbalances, thyroid disease, nutritional deficiencies, poor diet, magnesium deficiency, allergies, and prescription drugs like birth control pills, antibiotics, antihistamines, antiarthritis medications, and tranquilizers. Food allergies are one of the most common causes of depression.

Traditional therapies usually include counseling, psychiatric care, electroshock, and drug therapy. Special attention to the side effects of drug therapies must be researched, because side effects are many and varied. Be careful of what you take; research, and be thorough!

Natural therapies include dietary and nutrition changes; vitamins, supplements and herbal therapies; homeopathy; acupuncture; exercise; yoga; meditation; and self-hypnosis. Eating foods with the amino acid tryptophan increases serotonin in the brain, which eases tension. To promote alertness, eat high-protein foods to increase norepinephrine and dopamine.

Depression Relief Remedies

MENTAL ATTITUDE
Cause: suppression of goals or desires.
Cure: develop positive qualities and take action.

FOODS & DIET
Avoid: dairy products, alcohol, caffeine, sugar, salt, food colorings, preservatives, and additives, processed foods.
Good Foods: garlic, yogurt, watercress, turnips, soybeans, artichokes, beef, chicken, oat bran, sardines, endive, walnuts, salmon, mackerel, swordfish, kelp, molasses, lamb, coconut, liver, split peas, spinach, peas, bananas.

VITAMINS & SUPPLEMENTS
Multivitamin and mineral supplement with whole foods and enzymes, Vitamin C, B12, B complex, calcium, magnesium, choline, inositol, L-tyrosine, zinc, folic acid, chromium, EFA (essential fatty acids), GABA (gamma-aminobutyric acid), rutin.

HERBS
St. John's wort, oats, basil, ginkgo biloba, ginger, peppermint, ginseng, damiana, valerian, cumin, coriander.

AROMATHERAPY
Basil, jasmine, lavender, bergamot, patchouli, rose, geranium, sage, melissa.

The following scripts should be used in the morning and at night for at least six weeks. To optimize results, you may even want to try the scripts for anxiety, anger, fear and phobia, guilt, insomnia, and stress.

DEPRESSION SCRIPTS

THE CLOUD
Intention: To eliminate depression.

Find a comfortable place where you won't be disturbed, and sit in a comfortable chair. Now sit back and relax with both feet on the floor, and place your hands on the armrests of the chair or in your lap — whichever is comfortable for you.

Concentrate as you breathe deeply, letting the air come into your nose and out your mouth. Concentrate and breathe IN with the nose and OUT with the mouth. IN with the nose and OUT with the mouth. And IN with the nose and OUT with the mouth. Now let's concentrate on breathing OUT with the mouth and IN with the nose. And OUT with the mouth and IN with the nose. And OUT with the mouth and IN with the mouth.

Imagine that you are lying on a bed with clean, fresh, white sheets. It is the most comfortable bed and the sheets feel silky smooth against your skin. You seem to just sink down into this bed and you feel so safe and secure. You are so relaxed that you don't even have a care or worry in the world. Although you feel there is a lot of activity around you, you feel safe and secure just relaxing in the bed. You don't even have the desire to find out what is going on around you. You settle down into the soft bed and feel a deep, deep relaxation come over and into your body.

(Close your eyes for a moment and feel how relaxed you are.)

Touch the white sheets and as you do the bed turns into a big, white, soft, puffy cloud. You are so relaxed. You feel safe and secure. The cloud starts to rise and lifts you up out of the room into the most beautiful blue sky you have ever seen. Just feel yourself drift on this soft, white cloud which is raising you away from the world below. As the cloud rises, you feel all the chemicals in your body begin to balance. Shifting, changing, making you feel so centered and strong. You feel the changes taking place. You know that your mind, your body, your spirit are balancing to whatever is right for you to be happy and healthy.

(Close your eyes for a moment and feel the balance taking place.)

Look down over the edge of the cloud and see all the gloom below. Look up overhead and see the beautiful blue sky. See the sun shining brightly and feel it warm your body, taking away all the stress and tension that may be left in your body. The sun's rays are just melting all the stress, all the tension away from your body.

(Close your eyes for a moment and feel the stress leave your body.)

Feeling so relaxed and centered, watch as the sun's rays enter into your body, healing all your emotions and all your thoughts. Bringing everything into balance. Feel the shifts and changes taking place.

Watch as a beautiful rainbow appears above you. The colors are shimmering and brilliant in the sunshine. How beautiful it is. You feel very positive, joyful, happy. You feel whole and complete. What a wonderful feeling and you know that you are very, very special. You feel this joy and happiness in every bone, fiber, nerve, muscle, organ and in every thought in your body.

(Close your eyes for a moment and feel the joy and happiness.)

Watch as the bright lights of the rainbow start to flicker around you. You are filled with a sense of elation as the rainbow puts on a light show just for you. As the lights dance around before your eyes, you see your image in the colored lights. The image shows you how truly beautiful you are and how powerful you are. You feel, know, and trust who you truly are in this moment.

(Close your eyes for a moment and appreciate who you are.)

Joy starts to invade your body, your mind, your soul. You feel so powerful and you know you can cope with any situation. Feel the power! How whole and powerful you feel. Happiness and joy is your right and you feel these throughout your body. You know, feel, and trust that these feelings will stay with you.

THE ANGEL
Intention: To eliminate depression.

Find a comfortable place where you won't be disturbed, and sit in a comfortable chair. Now sit back and relax with both feet on the floor, and place your hands on the armrests of the chair or in your lap — whichever is comfortable for you.

Concentrate as you breathe deeply, letting the air come into your nose and out your mouth. Concentrate and breathe IN with the nose and OUT with the mouth. IN with the nose and OUT with the mouth. And IN with the nose and OUT with the mouth. Now let's concentrate on breathing OUT with the mouth and IN with the nose. And OUT with the mouth and IN with the nose. And OUT with the mouth and IN with the mouth.

Imagine you are walking in the rain. The clouds are dark and dreary. The rain is cold and wet. The landscape around you is in shadows. Look up at the sky to your left and you see a break in the clouds. Watch as the sun's rays seem to flicker through this break in the clouds. The clouds seem to dissipate and go away one by one as the sunlight becomes stronger. Before you is the biggest rainbow you have ever seen, and the beginning is right at your feet. The colors of the rainbow are so beautiful and the rainbow seems so solid. As you look closer at the rainbow, you see that it is really a bridge.

(Close your eyes for a moment and look at this rainbow bridge.)

The solid rays of beautiful light flicker as you start to walk up this beautiful bridge. As you take each step up the bridge, all your cares, all your worries just disappear. One by one.

(Close your eyes for a moment and feel the worry disappear.)

As you are nearing the top of the rainbow, an angel appears. The angel has the kindest and gentlest face you have ever seen. You sense a feeling of love for you as the angel motions for you to come closer. As you get closer to the angel, all your troubles and worries just melt away. The angel is smiling at you and you smile back. Now listen as the angel tells you everything you need to know to be well and happy. You may not be able to hear or understand the words, but that's okay, you know you are absorbing all the information that you need. You are getting information on how to be whole, healthy and happy.

(Close your eyes for a moment and listen to the angel.)

You feel the most tremendous peace come over your body. A feeling of serenity enters into your mind. Now watch as the angel touches the top of your head and a golden light surrounds you. You know that this angelic light is healing you. Making you whole and healthy right now. You feel the healing taking place.

(Close your eyes for a moment and feel the healing.)

When you are done healing, watch as the angel sends a feeling of pure love inside your mind, body, and spirit.

You feel the warmth of the love permeate your being. This pure feeling of love gives you happiness, joy, and peace.

Look up at the angel and smile. You know the angel will be there whenever you need anything. Feeling so very, very positive, say good-bye to the angel and walk back down the rainbow bridge. When you reach the bottom look up to the sky. You feel full of love, joy and happiness. You are centered and whole and you know this feeling will stay with you.

CHAPTER 18

Enlarged Prostate

The walnut-size, doughnut-shaped male sex gland called the prostate gland is located below the urinary bladder and surrounds the upper portion of the urethra. Through several ducts, prostate secretions or fluid pass into the urethra to increase transportation and nourishment of the sperm. Contraction of the muscles in the prostate squeezes the fluid, which makes up the bulk of semen, into the urethra.

Two common prostate problems are prostatitis and prostatic hypertrophy or enlarged prostate. Prostatitis is caused by infectious bacteria or hormonal changes, which cause inflammation of the prostate gland. This inflammation can cause urine retention, bladder infection, or kidney infection. Acute prostatitis symptoms are pain between the rectum and scrotum, frequent burning urination, fullness of the bladder, fever, chills, back pain, and blood in the urine. Chronic prostatitis symptoms can include frequent and burning urination, blood in the urine, lower back pain, and impotence, but the symptoms can be milder than in acute prostatitis.

Enlarged prostate (benign prostatic hypertrophy, or BPH) occurs in half of the men over 60 and three-quarters or more of the men over 70 years of age. Although the enlarged prostate of BPH is not cancerous, it can interfere with urination by obstructing the urethral canal, putting pressure on the kidneys, encouraging bladder infections, and creating frequent, burning urination and incontinence.

Bacteria, environmental chemicals (e.g., pesticides), tight underwear, and diet are some of the possible causes of enlarged prostate. Reducing cholesterol, hydrotherapy, drinking two quarts of water a day, avoiding exposure to cold weather, limiting over-the-counter cold and allergy medicines (which cause urinary retention and inflammation), and regular exercise (avoid bicycling) may help. Taking zinc and EFAs (essential fatty acids) daily may help prevent development of problems.

Typical treatment includes drug therapy. Check these drugs for side effects, which can include impotence, low libido, and hot flashes. Natural methods of treatment include: acupuncture, diet and lifestyle changes, herbal therapy, homeopathy, vitamin, mineral, and supplement therapy, visualization, and self-hypnosis.

Prostate Relief Remedies

MENTAL ATTITUDE

Cause: passivity.

Cure: initiate action and activity towards goals.

FOODS & DIET

Avoid: alcohol, tobacco, red meat, dairy products, sugar, carbonated drinks, caffeine, food colorings, additives, preservatives, processed meats, and other processed foods.

Good Foods: low-fat, high-fiber, mostly vegetarian diet, green tea, apples, broccoli, brown rice, cherries, cantaloupes, garlic, sesame seeds, lentils, carrots, cabbage, pumpkin seeds, chicken, soybeans, oatmeal, beets, spinach, walnuts, lamb, kelp, maitake mushroom.

VITAMINS & SUPPLEMENTS

Multivitamin and mineral supplement with whole foods and enzymes, Vitamin A, E, C, B complex, beta carotene, acidophilus, bioflavonoids, selenium, coenzyme Q10, zinc picolinate, L-cysteine, choline, folic acid, shark cartilage, L-carnitine.

HERBS

Saw palmetto, evening primrose oil, cumin, red clover, oat straw, buchu, damiana, stinging nettle, ginger, licorice root, echinacea, milk thistle.

AROMATHERAPY

Sage, tea tree, rose, jasmine.

The following scripts should be used in the morning and at night for at least six weeks. To optimize results, you may even want to try the scripts for general illness.

ENLARGED PROSTATE SCRIPTS

THE GOLD MINE

Intention: To eliminate enlarged prostate.

Find a comfortable place where you won't be disturbed, and sit in a comfortable chair. Now sit back and relax with both feet on the floor, and place your hands on the armrests of the chair or in your lap — whichever is comfortable for you.

Concentrate as you breathe deeply, letting the air come into your

nose and out your mouth. Concentrate and breathe IN with the nose and OUT with the mouth. IN with the nose and OUT with the mouth. And IN with the nose and OUT with the mouth. Now let's concentrate on breathing OUT with the mouth and IN with the nose. And OUT with the mouth and IN with the nose. And OUT with the mouth and IN with the mouth.

Imagine you are in a gold mine. The mine shaft that you are in is very, very dark. You have a miner's helmet on your head which has a light. As you look to your left you see a ladder going down deeper into the mine.

Go over to the ladder and start to climb down. With each step you feel more and more relaxed. You know this is a safe place and you have no fear.

(Close your eyes for a moment and feel how relaxed you are.)

As you climb down the ladder, look at the walls around you. They glisten as your light shines on them. When you reach the bottom of the ladder, turn around. There are two tunnels at the bottom here. One tunnel goes to your right and one goes to the left. Choose a tunnel and start to walk down it. Whatever tunnel you choose is the right one.

As you walk down the tunnel you see a large cavern. Stone is coming down from the ceilings and up from the floors in beautiful patterns. Look at these beautiful patterns of stone. The middle of the cavern is clear of all stones except for one right in the middle. Walk over to this stone. Leaning against the stone is a pick and a pail of liquid. You somehow know that embedded in this stone there is a walnut-sized piece of gold. Take up the pick and start carefully chipping away at the stone. Chip away the stone until you find the walnut-sized gold nugget.

(Close your eyes for a moment and chip at the stone.)

Watch as the stone surrounding the nugget gets smaller and smaller. The light from your helmet now shines on the gold nugget and it glistens and shines. Chip away the surrounding stone until the nugget becomes loose. There is debris of the stone you have chipped all around you.

(Close your eyes for a moment and see the nugget.)

Now pick up the pail of liquid. You know that this liquid is cleansing and healing. It will kill all the bacteria, the infection, and debris around the nugget. Pour the liquid on the gold nugget. Watch and feel how the nugget is being cleaned and healed. The nugget gets shiny as it reaches the original form that it was meant to be.

(Close your eyes for a moment and feel the healing taking place.)

The walnut-sized gold nugget is free of the surrounding stone. Pick it up and hold it in front of you. Look how it glistens and shines, just like brand new. Place the nugget in your pocket. At the side of the room there is a burlap bag and a shovel. Pick up the shovel and dig into the stone debris you have created. Place this debris in the burlap bag. Keep doing this until all the debris is in the bag. Now tie the bag with the rope that you find on the floor. Go back over to the ladder, bringing the burlap bag with you. Come out of the mine. When you reach the outside, throw the bag behind you.

Take out the nugget from your pocket and hold it up to the sun. It is so beautiful and it is exactly the right size for you. You feel happy and healthy, knowing you have done good work today, and you know that this feeling will stay with you.

THE ARMY
Intention: To eliminate enlarged prostate.

Find a comfortable place where you won't be disturbed, and sit in a comfortable chair. Now sit back and relax with both feet on the floor, and place your hands on the armrests of the chair or in your lap — whichever is comfortable for you.

Concentrate as you breathe deeply, letting the air come into your nose and out your mouth. Concentrate and breathe IN with the nose and OUT with the mouth. IN with the nose and OUT with the mouth. And IN with the nose and OUT with the mouth. Now let's concentrate on breathing OUT with the mouth and IN with the nose. And OUT with the mouth and IN with the nose. And OUT with the mouth and IN with the mouth.

Imagine you are lying in bed. You are relaxed and feeling very calm. Feel how each muscle in your body releases any tension it might have. Your neck, your back, your torso, your legs just release any tension that is there. You are so very, very relaxed.

Now imagine that inside your body you have a very small army with lots of soldiers. They are in tiny boats and they have magic guns. These guns shoot out healing light, and this light can heal your body. Watch as the soldiers steer their boats to any place in your body that has an infection. Feel the infection disappearing from your body as the soldiers shoot their guns with the healing light.

(Close your eyes for a moment and feel the healing.)

Now watch as the soldiers go to any area of your body that has any foreign bacteria. Watch them shoot the healing light and kill the bacteria wherever they are in your body. Healing your body. Making it whole and healthy.

(Close your eyes for a moment and feel the healing taking place now.)

Now watch as the soldiers go to any place that is enlarged in your body. Feel them shoot the healing light from their guns. As the light hits each spot, you feel how everything is shrinking, going back down to its original size. See how everything is becoming exactly the right size for you. You know this is happening in this time, in this place, right now.

(Close your eyes for a moment and feel the healing happening.)

Watch and feel how these soldiers, how your army is making you healthy and whole. Making everything work in correct and proper order. Continue to watch until you are completely healed. You feel happy, strong, relaxed and content. You know you are healthy and these feelings will stay with you.

CHAPTER 19

Fatigue

According to the dictionary, energy is internal or inherent power, potential force, or a capacity for vigorous action. Kinetic energy is the result of a body in motion. A person's energy can be affected by mental, physical, environmental, and spiritual forces. It is also affected by lifestyle, desires, and beliefs.

There are times when both men and women feel fatigue. Body fatigue is a symptom and not a disorder. Fatigue could be a warning signal of a health problem like chronic fatigue syndrome, poor circulation, allergies, *Candida,* poor food absorption, anemia, or a debilitating disease.

Fatigue can also be caused by boredom or depression. Everything is composed of energy. Remember that thoughts are also a form of energy. Being aware or conscious is energy in its most dynamic form. Negative thoughts and actions deplete energy, whereas positive thoughts or attitudes regenerate positive energy. The best way to utilize energy is to maintain a positive attitude and not to dwell on the negative. It has been proven that positive thought actually boosts the immune system and that negative thought depresses it. Remember: you are what you think.

Persistent fatigue that is not due to underlying physical causes or mental attitudes is usually the result of a poor diet, lifestyle, or inadequate rest. Nutrients provide food for the body, which turns into energy. Obtaining proper nutrients through diet, vitamins, and supplements helps the body and supports the mind to maintain energy. Adequate rest is important because when the body is at rest or sleeping, it is storing energy.

When someone is in need of extra energy, working with the whole person on a body, mind, and spirit level can help identify and eliminate the causes of fatigue. To maximize energy, a healthy lifestyle, diet, exercise, stress-reduction methods, and positive thought are required.

Natural methods for restoring or increasing energy include: acupuncture, aromatherapy, homeopathy, herbal therapy, vitamin therapy, exercise, tai chi, qi gong, yoga, meditation, visualization, and self-hypnosis.

Fatigue Relief Remedies

MENTAL ATTITUDE

Cause: fear of the results of goals and desires.

Cure: need to set goals and take action.

FOODS & DIET

Avoid: dairy products, alcohol, caffeine, sugar, salt, food coloring, preservatives, and additives, processed foods.

Good Foods: almonds, artichokes, beef, honey, cantaloupes, filberts, red peppers, grapefruit, eggs, chicken, rice bran, olive oil, grapes, tomatoes, watercress, lentils, peanuts, spinach, peas.

VITAMINS & SUPPLEMENTS

Multivitamin and mineral supplement with whole foods and enzymes, Vitamin C, E, B12, B complex, zinc, amino acids, pumpkinseed oil, bee pollen, cranberry, garlic.

HERBS

Wild oregano, Panax ginseng, rosemary, coriander, hawthorn, hops, kava, saw palmetto, tea tree.

AROMATHERAPY

Basil, lavender, bergamot, rose, neroli, sage, ylang ylang.

The following scripts should be used in the morning and at night for at least six weeks. To optimize results, you may even want to try the scripts for chronic fatigue and stress.

FATIGUE SCRIPTS

THE ATOMS
Intention: To increase energy.

Find a comfortable place where you won't be disturbed, and sit in a comfortable chair. Now sit back and relax with both feet on the floor, and place your hands on the armrests of the chair or in your lap — whichever is comfortable for you.

Concentrate as you breathe deeply, letting the air come into your nose and out your mouth. Concentrate and breathe IN with the nose and OUT with the mouth. IN with the nose and OUT with the mouth. And IN with the nose and OUT with the mouth. Now let's concentrate on breathing OUT with the mouth and IN with the nose. And

OUT with the mouth and IN with the nose. And OUT with the mouth and IN with the mouth.

Imagine you are in a tunnel. The tunnel is long and you can't see the end because there is very little light. Start walking down the tunnel. You feel safe and protected. At the back of the tunnel you begin to see lots of tiny flecks of bright light flashing. The tiny lights are moving quickly and flashing on and off.

(Close your eyes for a moment and see the lights.)

Walk towards the lights. As you get closer to the lights, you realize they are atoms of energy. The atoms of energy are moving quickly through the tunnel. Thousands and thousands of atoms are flickering their light on and off. Watch as these lights seem to flicker around you. Raise your right hand and hold it out with the palm up. Feel the energy of the atoms as they land in your palm.

(Close your eyes for a moment and feel the energy.)

Now watch as the energy is being absorbed within the palm of your hand. Your hand continues to absorb as much energy as you need. Watch and feel this energy filling your body. Giving your body all the energy it needs. Watch and feel this energy going into your mind, giving your mind all the energy it needs. Feel the energy coursing through your body, your mind. Making you powerful and strong. Giving you positive thought.

(Close your eyes for a moment and feel the energy within you.)

You are filled to the brim with all this positive energy. Feel how it sparkles within you. Feel the power inside you. Turn and walk out of the tunnel. As you walk out, you can feel the energy within you. You are happy and feel so energized, and you know this energy will stay with you.

OCEAN ENERGY
Intention: To increase energy.

Find a comfortable place where you won't be disturbed, and sit in a comfortable chair. Now sit back and relax with both feet on the floor, and place your hands on the armrests of the chair or in your lap — whichever is comfortable for you.

Concentrate as you breathe deeply, letting the air come into your nose and out your mouth. Concentrate and breathe IN with the nose and OUT with the mouth. IN with the nose and OUT with the mouth.

And IN with the nose and OUT with the mouth. Now let's concentrate on breathing OUT with the mouth and IN with the nose. And OUT with the mouth and IN with the nose. And OUT with the mouth and IN with the mouth.

Imagine you are walking near the ocean. It is right after a thunderstorm. The surf is coming in to the shore in huge, magnificent waves. Look at the colors in the ocean and the white curls of the waves. The sky is filled with sunlight that is bright and illuminating against the dark clouds. As you walk on the golden sand you can feel the energy in the air.

Find a spot that is comfortable for you and sit down on the sand, facing the ocean. Watch as the thundering waves come in to shore. Feel their power. The waves coming in and out as you sit relaxed on the sand.

(Close your eyes for a moment and look at the powerful waves.)

As you are watching the waves, you start to feel the air around you. It is so supercharged with energy. Take a deep breath and feel how this supercharged air goes into your body. Feel the air energizing your body as you breathe it in. Feel your body respond. It tingles with all this energy. Feel the energy going to every part of your body right now, in this time, in this place.

(Close your eyes for a moment and feel the energy in your body.)

Now take another deep breath and feel the supercharged air go into your mind. Feel it shift your mind, giving you energy, creativity, power. Feel the energy going to every part of your body right now, in this time, in this place.

(Close your eyes for a moment and feel the energy in your mind.)

Now take another deep breath and feel the supercharged air go into your spirit, your soul. Feel the shift in your spirit, giving you energy you need to manifest your purpose and who you are. Feel the energy going to every part of your spirit right now, in this time, in this place.

(Close your eyes for a moment and feel the energy in your spirit.)

You feel the most tremendous energy come over every part of you. Energizing your body, mind and spirit. Exhale and feel all the stagnation of your body, mind, and spirit as it just disappears.

Look out over the ocean and feel the energy of the ocean enter into your body and your mind. Continue to breathe as long as you need to. When you are done breathing, you feel you have all the energy you need. You know and you trust this, and this feeling will stay with you.

CHAPTER 20

Fear and Phobia

At the heart of disillusionment, anxiety, panic disorders, obsessive-compulsive disorders, stress, and phobias is a disease known as fear. All negative emotions are derived from fear. These emotions can encompass anger, frustration, embarrassment, denial, grief, envy, jealousy, insecurity, rage, resentment, stress, and worry.

Fear at its onset is a useful emotion because it exists in life as a means of protection, guidance, and as a way to get into action. Fear is the primitive fight or flight response that acts as a guidance system to protect and save your life. When there is a delay in taking action, or a refusal to face the fear, it no longer becomes useful, but is detrimental. At the point of non-action or refusal, fear intensifies and becomes prolonged. The symptoms of fear include: nausea; tightness in the chest, back, and neck; an uneasy mind; sweating; and rapid heartbeat.

There are many therapies and treatments for fear. They are all based upon the same premise: "Face your fear" or "Do what you fear." Facing fear transforms your mental attitude by increasing feelings of strength, self-worth, and control. Fear is definitely not a comfortable emotion, but by facing and transcending fear, this negative emotion is changed into a positive one.

Fear is not unlike the sensation of excitement. The same nerve endings in the body produce both emotions. What separates fear from excitement is the way you interpret it. Excitement creates acceptance in your mind and floods the body with interferons and interleukins, which are proteins that strengthen your immune system. Fear creates tension in your mind, which releases stress hormones in the body, which lower your immune system.

Irrational and rational fears stem from your belief system. Everyone fears unfamiliar situations, and fear will always be a part of life. However, 99% of fears are learned from what society has taught us, and most do not have a valid basis. Society also teaches that fear should be avoided, but you can reprogram your mind to welcome fear as your teacher.

There are four steps to managing fear and turning it into a positive emotion:

1. Acknowledge that the fear is there

2. Feel how the fear is affecting your body

3. Think about and determine what the best action is

4. Do the action.

Putting off the action results in delaying the release of the fear, which will stay until you release it. Facing fear is the only way to eliminate it. Natural methods for helping you deal with fear are counseling, aromatherapy, Bach flower remedies, meditation, visualization, and self-hypnosis.

Fear Relief Remedies

MENTAL ATTITUDE
Cause: refusal to investigate the unknown.
Cure: develop curiosity.

FOODS & DIET
Avoid: alcohol, caffeine, sugar, salt, food colorings, preservatives, and additives, drugs.
Good Foods: yogurt, protein foods, oat bran, turnips, watercress, oranges, strawberries, bananas.

VITAMINS & SUPPLEMENTS
Multivitamin and mineral supplement with whole foods and enzymes, Vitamin C, B1, B12, B complex, inositol, calcium, magnesium, chromium, phosphorus, potassium, zinc, manganese, niacin.

HERBS
Kava, oat straw, vervain, St. John's wort, lemon balm, hops, skullcap, linden flowers, wood betony, bilberry.

AROMATHERAPY
Rose, neroli, sandalwood, geranium, lavender, melissa, bergamot, jasmine, marjoram.

The following scripts should be used in the morning and at night for at least six weeks. To optimize results, you may even want to try the scripts for anxiety, low self-esteem, and stress.

FEAR AND PHOBIA SCRIPTS

THE DARK ROOM
Intention: To eliminate fear.

Find a comfortable place where you won't be disturbed, and sit in a comfortable chair. Now sit back and relax with both feet on the floor, and place your hands on the armrests of the chair or in your lap — whichever is comfortable for you.

Concentrate as you breathe deeply, letting the air come into your nose and out your mouth. Concentrate and breathe IN with the nose and OUT with the mouth. IN with the nose and OUT with the mouth. And IN with the nose and OUT with the mouth. Now let's concentrate on breathing OUT with the mouth and IN with the nose. And OUT with the mouth and IN with the nose. And OUT with the mouth and IN with the mouth.

Imagine you are in a hallway of a house with many rooms. The carpet is your favorite color and the pictures on the wall are beautiful. The hallway in front of you is very long. On both sides of the hallway is a series of closed doors. Feeling very relaxed and safe, walk down the hallway. There is a door to your right; open it and walk into the room. This room is the most beautiful room you have ever seen. All your favorite things are in this room and it feels so comfortable. How relaxed you feel here. How safe you are. How comfortable everything seems to be with all your favorite things around you.

(Close your eyes for a moment and picture this room.)

Walk out of this room and close the door. Walk to the end of the hallway. To your left you see a door; open it. Step into this room. The room is totally dark and you cannot see anything. You feel safe and now close the door behind you. Everything is dark and unfamiliar. You may even hear noises that you cannot identify. You may feel that the air is close around you. A small glimmer of light appears in the back of the room. The room starts to light up and you feel more relaxed. The light in the room grows brighter and brighter. As the room becomes light, you see many small tables crowded together side by side in the room. Look at the tables. On each table there is a different box. Walk over to a table that appeals to you. You are an observer and you know that in this place nothing can harm you. You feel safe and secure, more so than you have ever felt in your life. Open the box that is on that table that you selected. This box holds all your fears. Reach in the box and take out a fear and place it in the palm of your hand. Look at your fear. Turn it around and look at it from different angles and sides. Feeling very relaxed and calm, look at this fear.

(Close your eyes for a moment and look at the fear.)

You realize that this fear is very small. So small it fits in the palm of your hand. Look at the fear and place your ear next to it. Listen as the fear talks to you. It tells you what you need to do to reach your next step and how to release it. You may not hear the words but you know that you are getting all the information that you need. Listen as the fear tells you what action to take so it can be released. Ask the fear any questions you may have. The fear answers your questions with love, giving you all the information you need so it can be released.

(Close your eyes for a moment and listen to the fear.)

As you talk with the fear, you realize that the fear is your friend, your teacher. It wants to help you to be strong and centered. You feel your fear is giving you guidance and you know that the fear is giving you all the secrets on how to release it.

(Close your eyes for a moment and feel how the fear is your friend.)

Look at the fear and smile because you know that it is ready to be released. Hold the fear in the palm of your hand and say good-bye to it. Watch and hear the fear say good-bye to you. Now watch as the fear just disappears from the palm of your hand. You know you can come to this room at any time to face and talk to your fears so you can release them. You feel relaxed, centered, and self-empowered. You are ready to move on to the wonderful life that awaits you, filled with understanding and knowing. Close the box and walk out of the room. You are calm, relaxed, and filled with power, without a care or worry in the world, and this feeling will stay with you.

THE BEAR
Intention: To eliminate fear.

Find a comfortable place where you won't be disturbed, and sit in a comfortable chair. Now sit back and relax with both feet on the floor, and place your hands on the armrests of the chair or in your lap — whichever is comfortable for you.

Concentrate as you breathe deeply, letting the air come into your nose and out your mouth. Concentrate and breathe IN with the nose and OUT with the mouth. IN with the nose and OUT with the mouth. And IN with the nose and OUT with the mouth. Now let's concentrate on breathing OUT with the mouth and IN with the nose. And OUT with the mouth and IN with the nose. And OUT with the mouth and IN with the mouth.

Imagine you are in a forest. The trees are thick and very close to each other. You are walking on a path between the trees. Looking at the ground, you see many beautiful plants and interesting things. As you turn the corner in the path, you see a big bear standing in front of you. Your heart starts to quicken, your muscles get tense, but all of a sudden you begin to feel very, very calm. The closer the bear comes to you, the calmer you feel. This is a curious thing, but you cannot deny it because you feel so calm and relaxed. You notice that there is a light all around you. Look up and through the thick trees. You see a shaft of protective light falling from the sky, surrounding your body.

(Close your eyes for a moment and see this light.)

You know that this light is protecting you. It is guiding you to take the appropriate action. A knowing beyond words invades your body. You know what you are supposed to do. You feel calm and peaceful. Take the appropriate action now. You feel safe and secure. Calm and centered.

(Close your eyes for a moment and see yourself take the appropriate action.)

Look at the light coming in through the trees. How wonderful you feel. Now watch as the bear passes around you and out of sight. How centered and calm you feel. You know you will feel this way anytime fear comes into your life. You will feel calm, centered, and able to take the appropriate action. You trust in yourself to take the appropriate action. There is no doubt. Whatever action you take will be right for you. Feeling confident, in control, calm and relaxed, you know these feelings will stay with you.

THE MOONLIGHT
Intention: To eliminate fear.

Find a comfortable place where you won't be disturbed, and sit in a comfortable chair. Now sit back and relax with both feet on the floor, and place your hands on the armrests of the chair or in your lap — whichever is comfortable for you.

Concentrate as you breathe deeply, letting the air come into your nose and out your mouth. Concentrate and breathe IN with the nose and OUT with the mouth. IN with the nose and OUT with the mouth. And IN with the nose and OUT with the mouth. Now let's concentrate on breathing OUT with the mouth and IN with the nose. And OUT with the mouth and IN with the nose. And OUT with the mouth and IN with the mouth.

Imagine you are standing in the moonlight. Everything is dark around you, but the moon is shining the most beautiful soft light. You feel as if the moon is sending its beautiful light just around your body. You feel the glow of the moonlight all around you. This light is a protective light and you feel safe and secure in it. You are so relaxed with your body surrounded by this protective moonlight.

(Close your eyes for a moment and feel the moonlight.)

Now feel how this moonlight is giving you power over fear. Feel the moonlight enter into your mind and shift your mind to look at fear in a new way. You feel protected and fear cannot harm you. Feel the shift in your mind as your body stands in the moonlight.

The moonlight is bright and soft, yet it is so powerful around your body. Feel the moonlight go to your eyes. You know you can clearly see any messages that your fears want you to know. You are centered and safe, standing in the moonlight. Look at your fears through your new eyes.

(Close your eyes for a moment and look at your fears.)

You feel your mind and body shifting to want to handle any fear appropriately and quickly. You know you are thinking clearly without tension. Without stress. Feel the power that comes from within you. Feel the moonlight around you. You are always protected, safe, secure, in control, and you know you will take the appropriate action quickly to release your fears. This moonlight is magic and will stay around you, keeping your mind centered, positive, and powerful, and you know that these feelings will stay with you.

CHAPTER 21

General Illness

Illness and disease are caused by four types of stress: physical, emotional, nutritional, and environmental. Physical stress can be caused by a virus, germ, bacteria, parasite, fungus, infections, aging, or lack of exercise that causes your organs and body systems to work ineffectively. Emotional stress could include negative emotions (e.g., fear, anger), low self-esteem, resistance to future situations, and overall mental attitude. Examples of nutritional stress include improper diet, poor food absorption, and inadequate amounts of or lack of vitamins, supplements, amino acids, enzymes and other nutrients that your body needs to turn food into energy. Environmental stress happens through contact with hazardous chemicals, poisons, and outside pollutants (e.g., smog); over-the-counter, street, and prescription drugs; and excessive alcohol, tobacco, and other substance abuse. Repeated contact with environmental factors creates adverse chemical interactions, inside or outside the body, which result in the breaking down of the body.

The immune system is the body's defense against antigens or foreign substances that invade it. When a foreign substance initially invades the body, the immune system makes a memory of it. The next time the same foreign substance appears, the immune system uses this memory to fight the disease faster. Essential for survival, the immune system provides long-lasting immunity from disease.

The immune system watches the body's cells to make sure they are normal. Abnormal cells have a protein marker on their outer cell membranes that signals the immune system to destroy them. When the immune system spots a foreign substance in the body, it responds by producing two main types of lymphocytes that can destroy the abnormal cells. B cells are lymphocytes that produce antibodies and mature in the bone marrow. These antibodies circulate in the bloodstream and neutralize out-of-cell organisms such as bacteria, parasites, and viruses. T cells are lymphocytes that are responsible for the body's immunity; they mature in the thymus. Cytotoxic T cells directly kill organisms like bacteria and viruses that are inside infected cells. Helper T cells activate the cytotoxic T cells and B cells. There is another group of T cells called suppressor T cells, which slow down or stop T cell activity after infection has been eliminated.

Mature T and B cells circulate in the bloodstream and can also be found in secondary locations in the lymph nodes, lymphoid tissue, and spleen. These locations are where the immune system response begins. Aside from the T and B cells, there are larger lymphocytes that circulate in the blood but are found mostly in the spleen. These are called NK (natural killer) cells; they kill certain tumors and viruses. The part of the body where NK cells come from is unknown. The B, T, and NK cells are the essence of the immune system.

Aging can cause a natural decline of the immune system. Building up and maintaining a high-level immune system is the best way to combat disease and prevent illness. Controlling or eliminating the four types of stress keeps the immune system working at peak performance.

Treating the whole person and not specific symptoms improves immune system longevity and makes it work more effectively and efficiently. Lifestyle, the proper diet, vitamins, supplements, exercise, positive attitude and thought, and stress-reduction techniques all play an important role in boosting your immune system to maintain itself and work at top efficiency. Natural methods used to boost the immune system are acupuncture, homeopathy, Bach flower remedies, vitamins, supplements, herbal therapies, counseling, massage, meditation, visualization, and self-hypnosis.

General Illness Remedies

MENTAL ATTITUDE
Cause: denial of self.
Cure: self-acceptance and positive thinking.

FOODS & DIET
Avoid: wheat, white flour, white rice, all grains (except rye, corn, quinoa), cheese and dairy products (except eggs, butter, yogurt), meat (except lamb, chicken, turkey, venison, rabbit, duck), fermentation products, alcohol, vinegar, sugar, salt, carbonated drinks, coffee, caffeine, food colorings, preservatives, and additives, processed foods, citrus and all fruits (except tropical fruits), orange roughy, trout, oils (except flaxseed, safflower, olive, evening primrose, and borage), peanuts, macadamia nuts, yeast, iceberg lettuce, tomatoes, potatoes.
Good Foods: rye, corn, quinoa, oat bran, brown rice, wild rice, goat cheese, eggs, butter, yogurt, lamb, chicken, turkey, venison, duck, olive

oil, safflower oil, flaxseed oil, borage oil, evening primrose oil, sweet potatoes, yams, bananas, kiwi, pineapple, guava, papaya, avocados, pecans, strawberries, blueberries, beets, artichokes, cabbage, walnuts, cashews, almonds, vegetables, fish, royal jelly, spirulina, blue-green algae, kale, herbal teas.

VITAMINS & SUPPLEMENTS

Multivitamin and mineral supplement with whole foods and enzymes, Vitamin A, C, E, B complex, amino acids, enzymes, coenzyme Q10, DMG (dimethyl glycine), L-arginine, L-lysine, L-cysteine, bovine colostrum, acidophilus, NAC (N-acetyl cysteine), shark cartilage, melatonin, calcium, magnesium, beta carotene, bioflavonoids, pycnogenol, manganese, quercetin, selenium, chromium picolinate, lecithin, zinc.

HERBS

Garlic, cat's claw, melatonin, grape seed extract, pau d'arco, cumin, oregano, basil.

AROMATHERAPY

Sage, lavender, eucalyptus, rose, neroli.

The following scripts should be used in the morning and at night for at least six weeks. To optimize results, you may even want to try the scripts for chronic fatigue and stress.

GENERAL ILLNESS SCRIPTS

THE ANGELS
Intention: To eliminate illness.

Find a comfortable place where you won't be disturbed, and sit in a comfortable chair. Now sit back and relax with both feet on the floor, and place your hands on the armrests of the chair or in your lap — whichever is comfortable for you.

Concentrate as you breathe deeply, letting the air come into your nose and out your mouth. Concentrate and breathe IN with the nose and OUT with the mouth. IN with the nose and OUT with the mouth. And IN with the nose and OUT with the mouth. Now let's concentrate on breathing OUT with the mouth and IN with the nose. And OUT with the mouth and IN with the nose. And OUT with the mouth and IN with the mouth.

Imagine you are in a large open green field. The sun is shining and the sky is blue above you. Reach up your arms to the warm, golden sun. See your arms become long as they stretch towards the sun. Hold your palms out and feel the rays of the sun shine warmly into their center and then radiate out to your fingertips. Watch as individual rays of the sun touch each of your fingers. There are ten individual rays of sunlight reaching from the sun to your fingertips.

(Close your eyes for a moment and see these rays.)

Now watch as ten tiny angels walk down the rays of sunlight into the palm of your hand. These angels all have tiny lanterns of white light. You know these angels are here to heal you. Now watch and feel these ten tiny angels going into your body. Watch as they locate a trouble spot and hold up the lantern of white light to illuminate it. The light gets brighter at each trouble spot and heals it. Feel the healing light on each symptom.

(Close your eyes for a moment and feel how the light heals you.)

Now take some time and watch each of the ten angels healing you in all your trouble spots. One by one each trouble spot is disappearing in the healing white light, making you whole and perfect now.

(Close your eyes for a moment and watch the angels heal you.)

After the angels are finished, watch as the angels come out of your body the same way they went in. Now see the angels in the palms of your hand. They are smiling and you feel happy and healthy. Place the angels in your pocket. You know these are your own special healing angels that will help you whenever you need them. You are feeling very strong and healthy. You are relaxed and centered and you trust these feelings will stay with you.

WONDER HEALING*
Intention: To eliminate illness.

Find a comfortable place where you won't be disturbed, and sit in a comfortable chair. Now sit back and relax with both feet on the floor, and place your hands on the armrests of the chair or in your lap — whichever is comfortable for you.

This script is based on one used by hypnotist Steve Parker.

Concentrate as you breathe deeply, letting the air come into your nose and out your mouth. Concentrate and breathe IN with the nose and OUT with the mouth. IN with the nose and OUT with the mouth. And IN with the nose and OUT with the mouth. Now let's concentrate on breathing OUT with the mouth and IN with the nose. And OUT with the mouth and IN with the nose. And OUT with the mouth and IN with the mouth.

Imagine you are walking down a winding staircase into a secluded chamber. Notice the carpeting on the stairs — it is of an unusual texture. When you get to the bottom of the stairs you see a bookcase filled with very old books to your left. To your right you see a soft, comfortable chair with a light next to it. These books contain all the information that you need to heal yourself. Select a book and sit down in the chair. It doesn't matter which book you select — it is the right one for you. Turn on the light next to the chair and open the book. You may not be able to see the words, but that's okay, you know you are automatically absorbing all the information you need to heal yourself.

(Close your eyes for a moment and absorb the information.)

When you are done, replace the book in the bookshelf. Look to the back of the chamber; there is a door. Walk over to the door and go through it. This room has a television set with a big, comfortable sofa in front of it. Sit down on the sofa and feel how comfortable it is. Now watch as the TV screen turns itself on. On the screen you can see your illness. You know you are seeing inside all the parts of your body. Watch as the T cells, the B cells, and the natural killer cells come onto the screen. See how each kind of cells groups into a separate army. Watch as these cells go to each and every part of your body and attack the illness. Watch as these good cells drag all your illnesses off the screen, one by one by one.

You can feel the healing taking place in your body.

(Close your eyes for a moment, and the cells take your illness away.)

When you are done, look to the right of the room. There is a door there. Walk through the door.

In the middle of the room there is a table. The temperature in the room is just right for you. There is a chair in the room next to the table. Take off your clothes and put them on the chair. Now lie on the table on your back, face up. Look up over your head. You see a light there. Watch as the light turns into a beautiful emerald green.

You know that this light is a healing light. Watch as this light gets brighter and surrounds your body. Feel the emerald green light surround and go into your body. Feel the light healing any illness that is left inside your body, right now in this time, in this place. You can feel the healing taking place.

(Close your eyes for a moment and feel the healing.)

When you are done, you are happy. You feel healthy and you know you have done good work today. Now watch as the green light turns into a white light that surrounds your body. Protecting you from the illness. Giving you a sense of elation and well-being. You feel peace, happiness, and joy and you know these feelings will stay with you.

CHAPTER 22

Grief

Human beings form bonds of attachment throughout their lives. The attachment starts with their parents and then includes friends, significant others, intimate partners, and finally their own children. Disruption or loss of these bonds of attachment causes great mental pain, which is shown by grieving and mourning.

The grief process is normal. People never fully recover from losing someone they deeply love; they are changed by that loss. Hopefully, a new strength or other positive emotions are the result of that change. If the process of mourning does not take place, the grief may be delayed or show up in a negative way.

Abnormal grief, or pathological grief, is an intense and enduring response to the grieving process. Abnormal grief increases the risk of developing psychosomatic symptoms like illness, migraines, dizzy spells, anger episodes, and irritability. When a person is unwilling or unable to mourn, stress is maintained in the person's life until other life events help to bring the grief into focus.

The circumstances of the loss have an effect on the grief process. If the loss was unexpected or if a person had a highly dependent, attached, or love-hate relationship, there are higher risks for pathological grief.

The age of the person at the time of loss also has an effect on the grieving process. Each age handles death in different ways. Children may take grief in short doses, over different periods of time in their development process, until acceptance of the loss is finally reached. The elderly may have reached the acceptance level of their own life span and usually have been exposed to ever-increasing loss; therefore an elderly person will process grief much differently than a young child. Each stage of life has its own unique grieving process.

The normal initial reaction to loss is shock that it happened. The reality of the situation is then acknowledged. This is followed by a period of denial and then despair, which may include self-blame. Finally, detachment is realized and acceptance of the loss is obtained.

Spirituality can play an important role in helping to ease the grieving process. Thoughts of an afterlife can bring comfort to many in grief.

Acceptance that loss is part of the natural order of life can also aid grief. Throughout the ages, every culture has ways of dealing with grief, and all lead to the acceptance of the loss.

No matter what the age group or the circumstances surrounding the loss, there are five steps that can help the grieving process:

1. Accept the reality of the loss.

2. Experience the pain. Express the grief to family, friends, or a support group.

3. Honor the loss. Find a way to remember or commemorate the loved one.

4. Acknowledge and balance conflicting emotions. There will be both positive and negative emotions associated with the loss. Balance must be achieved so that the loss can be put into perspective. Bringing the facts of the relationship into awareness aids the mourner to achieve this balance.

5. Let go and move on. Letting go and saying good-bye on an emotional level allows the withdrawal of emotional investment in the loss. Restructuring the present and future is necessary for one to move on with life and participate in it.

Grief Relief Remedies

MENTAL ATTITUDE
Cause: lack of acceptance of life and death.
Cure: open up to spirituality.

FOODS & DIET
Avoid: alcohol, sugar, caffeine, food colorings, preservatives, and additives, processed foods.
Good Foods: yogurt, turkey, watercress, turnips, artichokes, avocados, oat bran, sardines, herbal teas.

VITAMINS & SUPPLEMENTS
Multivitamin and mineral supplement with whole foods and enzymes, Vitamin A, C, E, B complex, rutin, GABA (gamma-aminobutyric acid), EFA (essential fatty acids), L-tyrosine, choline, inositol, calcium, magnesium, zinc.

HERBS
Cumin, oregano, coriander, valerian, mugwort, gotu kola, lemon balm.

AROMATHERAPY
Hyssop, lavender, chamomile, rose, marjoram.

The following scripts should be used in the morning and at night for at least six weeks. To optimize results, you may even want to try the scripts for anger, anxiety, depression, and stress.

GRIEF SCRIPTS

THE BUTTERFLY
Intention: To eliminate grief.

Find a comfortable place where you won't be disturbed, and sit in a comfortable chair. Now sit back and relax with both feet on the floor, and place your hands on the armrests of the chair or in your lap — whichever is comfortable for you.

Concentrate as you breathe deeply, letting the air come into your nose and out your mouth. Concentrate and breathe IN with the nose and OUT with the mouth. IN with the nose and OUT with the mouth. And IN with the nose and OUT with the mouth. Now let's concentrate on breathing OUT with the mouth and IN with the nose. And OUT with the mouth and IN with the nose. And OUT with the mouth and IN with the mouth.

Imagine you are in a large meadow of flowers. Look at the green grass around you. Feel how soft and velvety it is to your touch. Look at all the beautiful flowers. There are so many pretty colors and they smell so good. The sky is blue and cloudless above you. The sun is shining and it is a perfect day. As you breathe in the scent of the flowers, your body begins to relax. Your mind becomes quiet. All your thoughts are at rest as you breathe in the wonderful scents of the flowers. Peaceful in this moment. If thoughts drift in, just let them drift away. You feel calm and centered, sitting here in this wonderful meadow of beautiful flowers.

(Close your eyes for a moment and feel how peaceful you are.)

Look down in front of you. You see the most wonderful flower you have ever seen. The color is bright and the smell is just right for you. Watch as a beautiful, delicate butterfly lands on the flower. Its wings are filled with soft, vibrant colors and they shine iridescently in the sun. All the colors in the butterfly's wings seem to vibrate with joy as it just sits on this flower in front of you. Everything is so perfect in this time and place. You feel a tremendous sense of love come up inside you. You are relaxed and calm, with this love soothing you, caressing you. You feel so safe and secure just watching this beautiful butterfly.

(Close your eyes for a moment and feel this love.)

Now watch as the butterfly goes away. You feel sad that it is going. It was so beautiful and you felt such love. You watch the butterfly as it goes away until you can no longer see it in the distance. Feel the emotions start to balance in your mind and your body. All the negative and positive emotions are coming into balance and perspective. Watch and feel your emotions balancing. Remember the beauty of the butterfly. You know and trust that you will always remember the beauty and love of that time with the butterfly.

(Close your eyes for a moment and feel and remember.)

Near you is a canvas, brushes, and paints. In this magic place you are a great artist. Make a picture of the butterfly. As you paint the picture, you see that the picture is perfect in every way. Through this picture the butterfly will always be part of your life. When you are done, look at the picture and feel all the love and beauty of the moment come back to you. This feeling will always be a part of you.

(Close your eyes for a moment and feel the feelings.)

Stand up and say a silent good-bye to the beautiful butterfly. Feel a gentle release come throughout your body. Look down at the beautiful flower and you know that other butterflies will land on this flower. Each butterfly is special and unique. Each one with its own special beauty. You know you will be back to see these butterflies and this brings you feelings of joy and love. Feeling relaxed, centered, filled with love, you know these feelings will stay with you.

THE HEART
Intention: To eliminate grief.

Find a comfortable place where you won't be disturbed, and sit in a comfortable chair. Now sit back and relax with both feet on the floor, and place your hands on the armrests of the chair or in your lap — whichever is comfortable for you.

Concentrate as you breathe deeply, letting the air come into your nose and out your mouth. Concentrate and breathe IN with the nose and OUT with the mouth. IN with the nose and OUT with the mouth. And IN with the nose and OUT with the mouth. Now let's concentrate on breathing OUT with the mouth and IN with the nose. And OUT with the mouth and IN with the nose. And OUT with the mouth and IN with the mouth.

Imagine you are in a safe place where no harm can come to your body. You are an observer and are just watching what is going on. Look inside your body. See that there are bands around your heart. Your heart is beating regularly and truly, at exactly the right pace for you. Now feel how the bands ever so slightly tighten around the heart. There is an emotional pain that comes from your feelings, and when the bands around the heart tighten, you feel this emotional pain. This emotional pain seems to be coming from within the heart and the bands are stopping the pain from releasing. Place your right hand over your heart and imagine a white light of energy coming out from the palm of your hand to your heart. Feel how warm and gentle this white light of energy is. Feel this energy enter your body and go around the heart. It is soft and warm and comforting.

(Close your eyes for a moment and feel this energy.)

Feel this energy melt the bands around your heart. Taking all the bands away from the heart. Each one disappearing, one by one. As each band disappears, you feel all the emotional pain release from your heart.

You feel lighter and you know the pain is going away.

(Close your eyes for a moment and feel the pain disappear.)

Now take your left hand and place it over your heart. Feel a golden light energy come out of the palm of your hand. Feel this golden light energy go into your heart. You feel a sense of love and healing permeating your heart, your mind, and your body. Your heart feels whole again. It is released from the pain and constriction. You feel open and free. Strong and alive. Feeling happiness and joy. You know these feelings will stay with you.

CHAPTER 23

Guilt

Guilt is described as a pervasive, destructive feeling of having to meet a high expectation or standard. Guilt is a mechanism that controls a person's behavior. It comes from the conscience, which defines the difference between right and wrong.

Guilt develops in childhood, from the expectation of reaching or matching a preconceived standard. The deepest sense of self, inherent values, and self-worth develop from the relationship of the parent and child. Parents and families hand down expectations to the young child, who has the need to be loved and to belong. If the parent or family sets limits with kindness, firmness, and teaches their children to acknowledge their feelings, they will instill appropriate guilt.

Appropriate or normal guilt acts as a helpful warning system that encourages the person to stay on the right track. In appropriate guilt, relief is gained by making amends for the negative action.

If the parent or family shames the child, gives mixed messages, doesn't set limits or follow through with limits, or sets unrealistic expectations, the child will have the feeling of being trapped and unlovable.

Debilitating guilt is caused by prolonged moral anxiety that is a vicious cycle. The guilt cycle starts with shame, which turns into anger. The anger creates anxiety, which brings in more guilt. This endless cycle establishes negative self-accusation, self-loathing, and unhappiness. In debilitating guilt there is no relief, even through punishment, making amends, self-punishment, or self-deprivation. Debilitating guilt is expressed in the mind, the body, and through actions. The mind reacts to guilt with negative self-talk and negative emotions such as sadness, disappointment, or anxiety. The body manifests debilitating guilt by showing symptoms of stress and fatigue. The stress and fatigue result in headaches, nervous disorders, and illness.

Actions stemming from debilitating guilt can include avoiding the guilt, overcompensating for the guilt, or losing control altogether.

Awareness of guilt and how it is processed in the person's emotions and life is helpful in resolving guilt issues. By changing the approach to guilt using self-respect, forgiveness, kindness, and love, guilt can be placed in its proper perspective.

There are four steps that can aid the release of guilt:

1. Listen to your feelings
2. Identify whether your guilt is appropriate or debilitating
3. Figure out how guilt can help you grow in a positive way
4. Take action.

Natural methods that can help alleviate guilt are counseling, Bach flower remedies, aromatherapy, meditation, visualization and self-hypnosis.

Guilt Relief Remedies

MENTAL ATTITUDE
Cause: attention on past mistakes or refusal to forgive.
Cure: find new approaches and take new actions.

FOODS & DIET
Avoid: alcohol, sugar, caffeine, food colorings, preservatives, and additives, processed foods.
Good Foods: yogurt, turkey, watercress, turnips, quinoa, artichokes, avocados, oat bran, sardines, soybeans.

VITAMINS & SUPPLEMENTS
Multivitamin and mineral supplement with whole foods and enzymes, Vitamin C, E, B12, B complex, bee pollen, zinc, calcium, magnesium.

HERBS
Panax ginseng, ginkgo biloba, basil, coriander, cumin.

AROMATHERAPY
Benzoin, frankincense.

The following scripts should be used in the morning and at night for at least six weeks. To optimize results, you may even want to try the scripts for anger, anxiety, depression, fear and phobia, and stress.

GUILT SCRIPTS

THE PICNIC
Intention: To eliminate guilt.

Find a comfortable place where you won't be disturbed, and sit in a comfortable chair. Now sit back and relax with both feet on the floor, and place your hands on the armrests of the chair or in your lap — whichever is comfortable for you.

Concentrate as you breathe deeply, letting the air come into your nose and out your mouth. Concentrate and breathe IN with the nose and OUT with the mouth. IN with the nose and OUT with the mouth. And IN with the nose and OUT with the mouth. Now let's concentrate on breathing OUT with the mouth and IN with the nose. And OUT with the mouth and IN with the nose. And OUT with the mouth and IN with the mouth.

Imagine you are in a picnic area. There is a family at the next table on your right with two children. They are cooking food and playing games. You are sitting at your picnic table. Look around to your left. There is a lake and the sun is shining off its surface. The summer air is balmy, yet a gentle breeze makes it just the right temperature for you. How peaceful you feel.

Watch as the family starts to play a game of baseball. The father is telling one of the children to hit the ball hard. The child hits the ball and it lands on your table, knocking over some of your food. Watch as the father yells at the child, calling him names. You are very uncomfortable at this.

(Close your eyes for a moment and feel how uncomfortable you are.)

The child begins to cry and the father now screams at the child to stop crying. Watch as the father tells the child to apologize to you. Look and feel the child's anxiety as he tries to run away. The father reaches out, catches the child. The father now drags the child over to your table. The child is stammering and crying as he offers you the apology. Feel how hurt the child feels. The shame and anxiety. Watch and feel how the guilt invades the child.

(Close your eyes for a moment and feel the child's guilt.)

Look up at the father and ask him to leave you alone with the child.

Ask the child to sit down. The child is nervous and anxious. Send the child a ray of love and warmth as you gently smile. Speak to the child with kindness and empathy. Assure the child he is forgiven.

(Close your eyes for a moment and talk to the child.)

Now let the child clean up the mess on your table. As the child cleans the table, walk over to the father and tell him whatever you need to. Feel love and kindness invade the air around you as you speak to the father.

(Close your eyes for a moment and feel the love around you.)

Watch as the child walks back to his table. There is peace and goodness surrounding everyone. Feel the self-confidence and value of everyone around you. The feeling of love is permeating every pore of your being and the entire family. This love is healing love. Everything around you is peaceful and in its proper order. Everything feels appropriate for you. Walk back to your table and sit down. You feel wonderful, happy, and have love all around you — and you know that these feelings will stay with you.

THE PARK BENCH
Intention: To eliminate guilt.

Find a comfortable place where you won't be disturbed, and sit in a comfortable chair. Now sit back and relax with both feet on the floor, and place your hands on the armrests of the chair or in your lap — whichever is comfortable for you.

Concentrate as you breathe deeply, letting the air come into your nose and out your mouth. Concentrate and breathe IN with the nose and OUT with the mouth. IN with the nose and OUT with the mouth. And IN with the nose and OUT with the mouth. Now let's concentrate on breathing OUT with the mouth and IN with the nose. And OUT with the mouth and IN with the nose. And OUT with the mouth and IN with the mouth.

Imagine you are in a magic city. All the beings are beautiful and they look so happy. The buildings are unusual and they are shining in the sun. Watch as people come up to you. They seem to know and like you very much. They talk and laugh with you and accept you for who you are. They have no expectations from you and they think you are wonderful. You feel very relaxed, happy, and stress-free.

(Close your eyes for a moment and feel how happy you are.)

Continue to walk through the city until you see a park with an empty bench. The bench is facing a beautiful lake. Sit down on the bench. Beautiful swans and rare birds are swimming in the lake and it is so peaceful here. Watch as a beautiful angel approaches you. Her truth and purity radiate white light all around her. Watch as she sits down on the bench next to you. She takes your hand and you feel pure love pour deep inside of you. Although the angel doesn't speak a word, you feel her tell you why you are so valuable.

She tells you how to develop your self-respect and how to identify your feelings and process them in the right way. Listen and hear what the angel is telling you. Listen as she tells you how to identify if any guilt is right or wrong and if it is appropriate for you. You feel a knowing happening in your mind as understanding comes into your being.

(Close your eyes for a moment and hear the angel.)

Now watch as she tells you how to forgive yourself and break the cycle of guilt step by step. Watch and listen as the angel tells you how to determine what actions you should take.

(Close your eyes for a moment and listen to the angel.)

Watch as the angel gets up from the bench, smiles at you, and leaves. You feel so peaceful and know that you can treat yourself with kindness. You know how special you are. Feel the love around you. You feel happy, self-confident, filled with freedom and joy, and you know that these feelings will stay with you.

CHAPTER 24

Headache

Headaches are one of the most common ailments. The main causes of headaches are fatigue, emotional disorders, and allergy. Brain tissue and the cranium (skull) cannot feel pain. Headache pain comes from the lining of the brain, cranial nerves, or the nerves of the upper neck. Ninety percent of headaches are tension headaches, which come from muscle tension and contraction. Tension headaches also are caused by improper ventilation, anxiety, depression, overwork, or worry. This type of headache is usually felt in the larger muscles of the neck and at the base of the shoulders and is brought on by muscle spasms in the neck and head. Tension headaches are aptly named, because they mirror the tension in your life. Eight percent of headaches are vascular headaches, known as migraines and cluster headaches. These are caused by the dilation of the blood vessels.

Sixty percent of migraine sufferers are women. Migraines usually develop between the ages of 10 and 30 years. This type of headache seems to cover one side of the head and skull. Migraines are usually accompanied by nausea; sometimes, there is distorted vision, fuzzy colored lights, numbness in the body, or an unpleasant odor preceding a migraine. Migraine headaches usually represent a state of anger; however, triggers for an attack can include PMS (premenstrual syndrome), drugs, fatigue, stress, birth control pills, and fasting.

Diet affects headache sufferers, especially those with migraines. Certain foods can trigger attacks. These include: cheese, chocolate, alcohol, MSG (monosodium glutamate), caffeine, food additives and dyes, processed meats, and nuts.

Cluster headaches, which often occur in males, produce severe, short pain attacks over one eye. These attacks can occur many times a day over a period of several months. These headaches usually involve an allergy symptom; for example, nasal congestion or a watery, teary eye.

The remaining 2% of headaches are the result of organic causes, such as sinus, eye, ear, nose, throat, and hypertension disorders.

Natural methods that can help people with headaches are acupuncture, aromatherapy, biofeedback, visualization, stress reduction, exercise, and self-hypnosis.

Headache Relief Remedies

MENTAL ATTITUDE
Cause: attention on past mistakes or refusal to forgive.
Cure: find new approaches and take new actions.

FOODS & DIET
Avoid: alcohol, sugar, caffeine, cheese, chocolates, soda, tea, food colorings, preservatives, and additives, MSG, bananas, eggplant, soy sauce, sour cream, processed meats and other processed foods.
Good Foods: garlic, grapefruit, fresh basil, almonds.

VITAMINS & SUPPLEMENTS
Multivitamin and mineral supplement with whole foods and enzymes; Vitamin C, E, B complex; bioflavonoids; bromelain; coenzyme Q10; quercetin; potassium, glucosamine sulfate; calcium; magnesium.

HERBS
Lavender, kava, ginger, skullcap, wood betony, lobelia, rosemary, St. John's wort, mint.

AROMATHERAPY
Rose, cardamom, chamomile, lavender, marjoram, rosemary, peppermint.

The following scripts should be used in the morning and at night for at least six weeks. To optimize results, you may even want to try the scripts for pain, depression, and stress.

HEADACHE SCRIPTS

THE DOG'S PAW
Intention: To eliminate headaches.

Find a comfortable place where you won't be disturbed, and sit in a comfortable chair. Now sit back and relax with both feet on the floor, and place your hands on the armrests of the chair or in your lap — whichever is comfortable for you.

Concentrate as you breathe deeply, letting the air come into your nose and out your mouth. Concentrate and breathe IN with the nose and OUT with the mouth. IN with the nose and OUT with the mouth. And IN with the nose and OUT with the mouth. Now let's concentrate on breathing OUT with the mouth and IN with the nose. And OUT with the mouth and IN with the nose. And OUT with the mouth and IN with the mouth.

Imagine you are in sitting in a veterinarian's office. Look around and see the counter. Look at the dogs and cats sitting in the waiting room. They are waiting to see the vet. Look to your left and see a cute dog with a bandage around its paw. Look closer at the paw and see how tight the bandage is. The bandage is so very, very tight. You can see the paw pulsating where the bandage does not cover the dog's toes. Look at the dog's face and see the pain in its eyes. Feel the aching in the dog's paw.

(Close your eyes for a moment and feel how the dog paw feels.)

Look to your right and you see the vet coming out of a room. The vet is smiling. Watch as he greets the dog with the bandaged paw by talking to it soothingly and patting it on the head gently. Watch as the vet picks up the dog and brings him to a back room. Follow the vet into the back room. Listen as the vet tells the dog that everything is going to be all right. Now watch as the vet starts to unbandage the dog's paw. There is no blood. You can see the relief in the dog's eyes as the blood starts flowing freely inside the paw. The area once covered by the tight bandage is completely free and open now as the vet throws the bandage on the floor. Feel the tingle and relief as the blood continues to flow freely inside the paw. All the pain is gone. Feel the dog healing. As you watch the dog, you feel your own pain just melting away. You are free from pain. Your blood is flowing freely without restriction. All your muscles in your neck and shoulders are so relaxed. Feel the pain just going away.

(Close your eyes for a moment and feel your pain just going away.)

Now watch as the dog becomes happy because it is pain-free. You are so relaxed and happy. Your pain is completely gone and you feel whole and healthy, and you know that this feeling will stay with you.

THE AURA
Intention: To eliminate headaches.

Find a comfortable place where you won't be disturbed, and sit in a comfortable chair. Now sit back and relax with both feet on the floor, and place your hands on the armrests of the chair or in your lap — whichever is comfortable for you.

Concentrate as you breathe deeply, letting the air come into your nose and out your mouth. Concentrate and breathe IN with the nose and OUT with the mouth. IN with the nose and OUT with the mouth. And IN with the nose and OUT with the mouth. Now let's concentrate on breathing OUT with the mouth and IN with the nose. And OUT with the mouth and IN with the nose. And OUT with the mouth and IN with the mouth.

Imagine yourself floating on a cloud. The clouds are soft and fluffy around you. You are so relaxed and comfortable as all the tension, all the stress just seems to leave your body. All your muscles are relaxing in this soft, soft cloud. All your thoughts just drift away until you are very relaxed and peaceful without a care or worry in the world. Imagine that there is a red light in your aura around your head. It is very, very bright. This red light seems to be surrounding your head.

(Close your eyes for a moment and see this red light.)

Look up to the sun and see a blue ray of light come out of the sun and watch as it surrounds your head. It is the most beautiful blue you have ever seen. You feel very calm and centered with this blue light surrounding your head. Watch as the blue light infiltrates and diffuses the red light that surrounds your head. Watch as all the red disappears and only the soft, gentle blue light is in your aura. As this is happening, feel your headache pain just disappear.

(Close your eyes for a moment and feel the blue light.)

The blue light feels cool and light, yet warm and soothing all at the same time. Feel the healing taking place within your head, your neck, your shoulders. Feel the pain just going away. Watch as the blue light reaches every nook and cranny inside your head. You are pain-free, peaceful, and so relaxed, and you know that these feelings will stay with you.

CHAPTER 25

High Blood Pressure

High blood pressure is also known as hypertension. The heart pumps blood through the arteries in the body. This pumping of the blood causes a pressure on the blood vessel walls. When this pressure is high, it is called high blood pressure.

Fluctuating blood pressure is normal; blood pressure increases with emotional stress, physical activity, fear, or excitement. However, consistent high blood pressure is not normal. The output of blood from the heart, resistance of flow through the blood vessels, the amount of blood, and how it is distributed to the organs of the body determine high or low blood pressure. Physically, high blood pressure is usually caused by an increased blood flow from the heart that cannot pass through the artery branches called arterioles.

High blood pressure is placed in two categories: primary or secondary. Primary high blood pressure can be caused by genetics, alcohol, obesity, emotional stress, inactivity, excessive salt in the diet, birth control pills, and water retention. It can also be caused by overactivity of the sympathetic nervous system in the body, which controls the heartbeat rate, its force, and the tone of the arterioles and veins. Secondary high blood pressure is the result of underlying health problems such as kidney or adrenal gland disorders and disease.

Blood pressure can rise when arteries have been damaged by excessive fat, oil, and cholesterol in the diet. The arteries begin to close up. If increased salt is in the diet, this attracts more fluid into the bloodstream and blood pressure increases through the already impaired arteries. High blood pressure can accelerate arteriosclerosis or hardening of the arteries, as well as making target organs such as the heart, brain, kidneys and eyes vulnerable.

Transformation of lifestyle is the key to controlling high blood pressure. To prevent or control high blood pressure, try to eat a low-fat, high-fiber, salt- and alcohol-free diet; lose excess weight; take the right supplements; exercise; and use relaxation methods. Healing and wellness retreat centers that provide juice fasting, cleansing, and dietary programs can support lifestyle changes that culminate in lowering high blood pressure.

High Blood Pressure Relief Remedies

MENTAL ATTITUDE

Cause: feelings and attitudes of overresponsibility.

Cure: develop purpose and learn to compete with the self and not others.

FOODS & DIET

Avoid: white flour, sugar, salt, alcohol, caffeine, junk food, nicotine, artificial flavorings, colors, preservatives.

Good Foods: squash, avocado, cantaloupe, eggs, grapes, flaxseed oil, borage oil, black currant oil.

VITAMINS & SUPPLEMENTS

Multivitamin and mineral supplement with whole foods and enzymes, Vitamin C, B6, L-glutamine, selenium, L-carnitine, niacin, zinc, melatonin, calcium, magnesium, potassium, chromium, beta carotene, coenzyme Q10.

HERBS

Dill, parsley, garlic, yarrow, hawthorn, wood betony, linden flowers.

AROMATHERAPY

Lavender, rose, neroli.

The following scripts should be used in the morning and at night for at least six weeks. To optimize results, you may even want to try the scripts for general illness and stress.

HIGH BLOOD PRESSURE SCRIPTS

THE GARDEN HOSE

Intention: To reduce high blood pressure.

Find a comfortable place where you won't be disturbed, and sit in a comfortable chair. Now sit back and relax with both feet on the floor, and place your hands on the armrests of the chair or in your lap — whichever is comfortable for you.

Concentrate as you breathe deeply, letting the air come into your nose and out your mouth. Concentrate and breathe IN with the nose and OUT with the mouth. IN with the nose and OUT with the mouth. And IN with the nose and OUT with the mouth. Now let's concentrate on breathing OUT with the mouth and IN with the nose. And OUT with the mouth and IN with the nose. And OUT with the mouth and IN with the mouth.

Imagine you are in a garden. It is so beautiful here with all the colors and wonderful smells. Listen to the birds singing; how peaceful it is here. The sun is shining and the temperature of the air is exactly right for you. It is relaxing here in the garden with no pressure or stress. Everything is so very serene and peaceful.

(Close your eyes for a moment and feel the peace of the garden.)

As you look at the plants in the garden, you realize that they need to be watered. Look to your left. You see a faucet with a garden hose attached. Turn on the faucet and pick up the hose. The water is coming out of the hose very fast. The pressure of the water makes the hose start to slip out of your hands. Hold onto the hose tightly. You are in control. Watch as the pressure of the water hits the plants and flowers. The pressure of the water makes the plants and flowers fall over. Turn back to the faucet and adjust it to lower the pressure. The faucet seems stuck. You cannot turn it. The water from the hose is out of control. Kneel down near the faucet. Breathe in deeply and evenly and blow the air out of your mouth towards the faucet. Continue breathing in evenly, deeply, rhythmically and blowing out your air towards the faucet. As your air hits the faucet, watch how the water is slowing down out of the hose. Continue blowing towards the faucet in a steady, even rhythm until you see the water from the hose flowing slowly with steady, even pressure. Flowing in the exact amount that is right for you.

(Close your eyes for a moment and see the flowing water.)

Now watch as the water flows freely, evenly, with just the right pressure. Everything is in good working order. Water the plants and the flowers. Watch as the water flows gently and evenly in just the right pressure from the hose. Go over to the faucet and turn off the water. Now turn the water back on. The pressure is steady and even. Rhythmic. You have fixed the problem and are very happy. Look at the flowers and plants in the garden. They are so beautiful and healthy. Everything is so peaceful and serene. You are feeling so relaxed and stress-free.

(Close your eyes for a moment and feel how relaxed you are.)

Look to your right. There is a bench in the garden. Go over to the bench and sit down. The bench is dry from the sun. Close your eyes and just relax. Feel the sun on your body. Feel the rays permeating through your body. Each ray relaxing you, taking away all your stress. Feel the sun's rays enter into your body. Now feel the rays adjusting your body, your heartbeat, the force of your blood flowing through your body, making everything exactly right for you. Adjusting all the systems in your body until they are working correctly, as you just sit in the sun relaxing without a care or worry in the world. Feel this gentle adjustment to your body.

(Close your eyes for a moment and feel your body healing.)

You know your body is working exactly right for you. You feel so relaxed and peaceful. This feeling will stay with you.

THE HEALING CHAIR
Intention: To reduce high blood pressure.

Find a comfortable place where you won't be disturbed, and sit in a comfortable chair. Now sit back and relax with both feet on the floor, and place your hands on the armrests of the chair or in your lap — whichever is comfortable for you.

Concentrate as you breathe deeply, letting the air come into your nose and out your mouth. Concentrate and breathe IN with the nose and OUT with the mouth. IN with the nose and OUT with the mouth. And IN with the nose and OUT with the mouth. Now let's concentrate on breathing OUT with the mouth and IN with the nose. And OUT with the mouth and IN with the nose. And OUT with the mouth and IN with the mouth.

Imagine you are sitting in the most comfortable chair. You are relaxed and as you look around the room you see nothing but white walls, a white ceiling, and a white floor. The only color in the room is the chair you are sitting in. The chair's fabric is in your most favorite color and pattern. As you look at the bare white walls, all thoughts from your mind just disappear. You are just relaxing, just being here in this moment.

Now let your mind go back to a time when you felt happy and healthy. Let your mind drift back to a time when your blood pressure was normal and working exactly right for you. Feel how you felt at that time. Feel how your heart is beating in rhythmic, regular heart beats. How your arteries were letting the blood flow evenly at the correct pressure through your body. Remember this time. Feel how healthy your body is. Feel how the blood flows freely and evenly to your organs and throughout your body. Feel how happy and stress-free you are.

(Close your eyes for a moment and imagine this time.)

Now feel how your body is responding to that memory. Your blood pressure getting even and steady, just right for your body. Feel your heart beating regularly as your body remembers and adjusts itself to work exactly right for you. The blood flowing evenly with just the right amount of pressure to your organs and throughout your entire body. You feel your body working correctly.

(Close your eyes for a moment and feel your body adjusting.)

You know that your body will continue to do this. You trust that your blood pressure is normal and will continue to be normal, working exactly right for you. You are so relaxed and happy. This feeling will stay with you.

CHAPTER 26

Impotence

Impotence or erectile dysfunction means that a man does not have the ability to achieve or maintain an erection adequate for sexual intercourse. Erections come from brain stimuli, nerve and blood vessel function, and hormonal activity. The myth that most impotence comes from a psychological basis is not true. The facts are that 85% of impotence results from a physical problem. Chronological age is not as much of a factor as the aging process itself. With proper diet, exercise, and stress reduction, your physical body can be much younger than your chronological age.

Most males will experience occasional episodes of impotence from fatigue, excess alcohol intake, or distress. Some of the signs of physical impotence are: if your sexual performance has deteriorated over time, you are not having erections during sleep, or you cannot maintain an erection during masturbation. The causes of physical impotence are: vascular disease, hardening of the arteries, heart disease, hormone imbalances, hypertension, nerve damage, pelvic trauma, and radiation treatment. Prescription and over-the-counter drugs can account for impotence. Over 200 drugs have been identified as possible causes, including: alcohol, nicotine, stomach acid inhibitors, and ulcer medications. Seeking the help of a qualified doctor can help determine the physical cause.

Some of the signs of psychological impotence are: sudden loss of potency, death of a loved one, a life crisis, if you can have sex with some partners and not others, and if during masturbation you can maintain an erection. The causes of psychological impotence can include: performance anxiety, low self-esteem, marital discord, guilt, sexual abuse, and depression. Seeking the help of a qualified counselor may help in these situations.

There are four stages of impotence: 1) denial, rationalization, and hope; 2) depression, anger, and fear; 3) exploration of the causes; and 4) making a decision on what to do about it.

There are many therapies and alternatives for impotence, such as aphrodisiacs, medical injections, drug therapy (research shows long-term side effects are possible), and external and internal devices (e.g., penile implants).

Natural methods that can help are acupuncture, change of diet and lifestyle, vitamin and supplement therapy, exercise, herbal therapies, homeopathy, Bach flower remedies, stress-reduction techniques, visualization, and self-hypnosis.

Impotence Relief Remedies

MENTAL ATTITUDE
Cause: fear of results of goals and desires.
Cure: need to set goals and take action.

FOODS & DIET
Avoid: alcohol, sugar, caffeine, food colorings, additives, preservatives; processed meats and other processed foods.
Good Foods: garlic, grapefruit, fresh basil, almonds.

VITAMINS & SUPPLEMENTS
Multivitamin and mineral supplement with whole foods and enzymes, Vitamin A, E, B complex, zinc, DMG (dimethyl glycine), octacosanol, L-tyrosine.

HERBS
Wild yam, cumin, ginseng, damiana, sarsaparilla.

AROMATHERAPY
Lavender, rose, patchouli, sage, ylang ylang.

The following scripts should be used in the morning and at night for at least six weeks. To optimize results, you may even want to try the scripts for self-esteem, guilt, depression, stress, and general illness.

IMPOTENCE SCRIPTS

THE PERFECT CAR
Intention: To eliminate impotence.

Find a comfortable place where you won't be disturbed, and sit in a comfortable chair. Now sit back and relax with both feet on the floor, and place your hands on the armrests of the chair or in your lap — whichever is comfortable for you.

Concentrate as you breathe deeply, letting the air come into your nose and out your mouth. Concentrate and breathe IN with the nose and OUT with the mouth. IN with the nose and OUT with the mouth. And IN with the nose and OUT with the mouth. Now let's concentrate on breathing OUT with the mouth and IN with the nose. And OUT with the mouth and IN with the nose. And OUT with the mouth and IN with the mouth.

Imagine you are standing in front of a car. The car is your favorite color and the inside of the car is so luxurious. Look at the outside of the car. It looks sleek and fast. The sun glints off the hood. Get into the car and sit behind the wheel. Smell the leather. Feel the dashboard. This is the car you have always wanted. It is hot and beautiful. The keys are in the ignition; turn the car on. It is running evenly and smoothly. Rev up the motor. You feel so powerful just sitting in the car without a care or a worry in the world.

Take the car out onto the road. It handles exactly as you want it to handle. There is a long, straight country road ahead of you. Step on the gas. Feel the gas going into the engine, giving the car power. You know that the engine is getting the power it needs. The gas is flowing into the engine. Filling the engine. Giving the engine the power it needs to go faster. Step on the gas and feel the car go forward.

(Close your eyes for a moment and feel how powerful the engine is.)

This is a magic car. No matter how long you drive, the gas tank is always full. The gas is always able to feed the engine, making the car powerful and strong. Thrusting the car forward. You know that the car will always work the way you want it to, without effort, without worry. Look to the right; you see a beautiful place to pull the car over. Park the car. Get out of the car and look at the view. It is the most beautiful view you have ever seen. The sun is shining and the outside temperature is exactly right for you. All your stress, all your tension seems to just go out of your body.

(Close your eyes for a moment and feel the stress leave your body.)

Now look up to the sun and feel the sun's rays enter into your body. The rays are warm and soothing. As the rays enter your body, you feel strong. You know that the rays are healing anything in your body that needs healing. The rays are making your body strong and healthy, able to perform. Feel the rays healing your body in this time, in this place, right now.

(Close your eyes for a moment and feel the healing taking place.)

Feel the sun's rays enter into your mind, your nerves, your blood vessels, your hormonal glands. Feel the rays healing and balancing all these areas. Feel the healing taking place now.

(Close your eyes for a moment and feel the healing taking place.)

Now watch and feel the sun's rays come out of your body the same way they went in. Watch as the rays take with them anything that has stopped you from your performance. All the thoughts, all the physical problems are leaving your body. Leaving you strong, whole, and balanced.

(Close your eyes for a moment and watch the rays come out of your body.)

Walk over to the car and get back in. Start the car and step on the gas. Feel how the gas goes into the engine, freely without obstruction. Watch as the engine receives the gas and propels the car with power. The car is strong and powerful, just as you are. As you drive the car down the road, feel how in control you are, how powerful, healthy, and strong you feel, and you know that everything is in top working order. This feeling will stay with you.

THE BICYCLE
Intention: To eliminate impotence.

Find a comfortable place where you won't be disturbed, and sit in a comfortable chair. Now sit back and relax with both feet on the floor, and place your hands on the armrests of the chair or in your lap — whichever is comfortable for you.

Concentrate as you breathe deeply, letting the air come into your nose and out your mouth. Concentrate and breathe IN with the nose and OUT with the mouth. IN with the nose and OUT with the mouth. And IN with the nose and OUT with the mouth. Now let's concentrate on breathing OUT with the mouth and IN with the nose. And OUT with the mouth and IN with the nose. And OUT with the mouth and IN with the mouth.

Imagine you are riding a bicycle. It is a beautiful summer day. The sun is shining and a few wispy clouds are in the sky. You have no commitments, no cares, no worries. Feel how relaxed and peaceful you are as you pump your legs and ride the bicycle.

Look at the scenery around you. How nice this is. Just in front of you there is a steep hill. The hill is the biggest you have ever seen. Look down at the ground to your right. There is a golden coin glinting in the dirt. Stop the bicycle and reach down and pick up the coin.

The coin is very old and you have not seen one like it before. Place the coin in your right hand. Now watch as a healing light comes out of the coin and fills your body. Feel this golden light enter into your body and your mind.

(Close your eyes for a moment and feel the light.)

The light is making you strong and powerful. You feel this energy enter into your body. All doubt seems to just disappear as you hold this golden coin in the palm of your hand.

(Close your eyes for a moment and feel the doubt just disappear.)

Look at the coin. Feel the power. Now place the coin in your pocket. You know that the coin's light has made you strong and powerful. Look up at the steep hill and start riding your bicycle.

You feel so powerful as you thrust forward, propelling the bicycle up the hill. The closer you come to the top, the stronger you feel. The energy is flowing through your body. You feel and know this. The more you pump your legs, the more power you feel. You are coming closer and closer to the top. You feel strong. All your muscles in your body are working at top capacity. Filled with energy and power. All your body in perfect working order.

(Close your eyes for a moment and feel your energy and power.)

When you reach the top, look back down the hill. You have conquered your problem. You have reached the top of the hill. Look down the hill and watch as the hill disappears and becomes a flat, even path. You have conquered the hill and your body feels powerful, strong, and filled with energy. You can conquer anything! You feel positive and happy and you know that this power, this strength, and this energy will stay with you.

CHAPTER 27

Infertility and In Vitro Fertilization

Infertility. Infertility is usually defined as the inability to conceive after twelve months of unprotected intercourse during the time of ovulation, whether it is in the attempted conception of a first child or after the successful birth of a child.

For women, the intricate process of ovulation, fertilization, the fertilized ovum's journey through the fallopian tubes and its attachment in the uterus must all work perfectly for a pregnancy to occur.

The overall causes of infertility are as follows: a problem of the male partner's, tubal damage, ovulatory problems, endometriosis, and unexplained problems.

Males are responsible for approximately 25% of infertility. Tubal damage can stem from infection, sexually transmitted diseases, appendicitis, and abdominal surgery. Ovulation problems include blocked, defective, or failed ovaries; cysts; egg retention; elderly eggs; drugs; and smoking. Endometriosis results when fragments of the uterine lining are in other places, usually in the pelvic cavity. Uterine fibroids are also a potential problem. Infertility could be caused by emotional factors (e.g., stress and fear), obesity, being underweight, alcohol, caffeine, drugs, or heavy metal poisoning.

For men, infertility can be caused by deficient sperm or an anatomical abnormality. Sperm may be deficient in a number of ways, including low sperm production, impaired sperm mobility, and sperm head shape. Sperm are produced on average at a rate of 1800 per second from each testicle at an average count of 100 million per milliliter. Counts below 20 to 40 million per milliliter are considered subfertile or below normal. Anatomical abnormalities could include a dilated vein in the spermatic cord, varicose veins in the testes, and delayed descent of the testes.

Some of the causes of male infertility are: genetic problems, exposure to toxins and radiation, endocrine disorders, mumps, sexually transmitted diseases, alcohol, drugs, testicular injury, blockage of the vas deferens, and tight clothing.

Fertility drugs such as clomiphene citrate (marketed as Clomid and Serophene), gonadotropins, and bromocriptine stimulate the growth of follicles of the ovary. They are normally given to women who have failed or limited ovulation. Side effects of these drugs can include: ovarian enlargement, blurry vision, skin rashes, hot flashes, ovarian cancer, abdominal pain, cramping, cervical mucous membrane abnormalities, miscarriage, multiple gestation, nausea, and dizziness.

A healthy diet, vitamins, supplements, exercise, and correct body weight can help. For both men and women, avoiding cow's milk (which is high in estrogens), soy products, and environmental chemicals like insecticides can increase your chances of fertility. Emotional support is also important. Don't isolate yourself by avoiding family or occasions where children are present. Share the burden with friends, family, or a support group. Remember to keep positive – miracles happen every day.

Natural therapies include acupuncture, aromatherapy, Bach flower remedies, homeopathy, reflexology, relaxation, and self-hypnosis.

In vitro fertilization (IVF). In vitro fertilization is a combination of fertility drug therapy with the surgical assistance of embryo transfer procedures to improve conception. In the United Kingdom ART (assisted reproductive techniques), which encompass IVF, are well regulated, their success rates are published, and clinics are not allowed to place more than three embryos in a woman. In the United States, regulation is voluntary.

If a woman has no fallopian tubes, in vitro fertilization is her only answer for conception. The procedure usually consists of placing a woman on drugs to create artificial and temporary menopause, in which the effects can last from a few days to four weeks. Then an injection is given to stimulate the growth of several follicles. Normally just one egg is produced at a time, but these follicles will produce multiple eggs. When the follicles are mature enough, another injection is given, and approximately 35 hours later, the eggs are collected.

At the time the eggs are collected, a semen sample is provided by the male partner. This semen sample is prepared to be used in the fertilization process.

The eggs and sperm are placed in a petri dish, and fertilization takes place within the next 24 to 48 hours. Then the fertilized eggs are implanted by a catheter into the woman's uterus, and natural implantation takes between 5 to 7 days. Pregnancy can be confirmed 10 to 14 days later. This method has a success rate for full-term pregnancy of approximately 20%.

GIFT (gamete intra-fallopian transfer), IUI (intrauterine insemination), ZIFT (zygote intra-fallopian transfer), TET (tubal embryo transfer), PROST (pronuclear-stage transfer), and POST (peritoneal oocycle sperm transfer) are similar or refined methods of in vitro fertilization.

Proper diet, lifestyle, weight management, nutrients, vitamins, and supplements, and self-hypnosis can help.

Infertility Relief Remedies and Remedies to Aid In Vitro Fertiliation

MENTAL ATTITUDE

Cause: insecurity.

Cure: develop initiative and believe.

FOODS & DIET

Avoid: alcohol, sugar, caffeine, cow's milk, soybeans, food coloring, additives, and preservatives; processed meats and other processed foods.

Good Foods: elderberries, parsley, guava, rose hips, squash, romaine, almonds, spinach, asparagus, broccoli, molasses, maple syrup, egg yolks, brown rice, lentils, peas, liver, royal jelly.

VITAMINS & SUPPLEMENTS

Multivitamin and mineral supplement with whole foods and enzymes, Vitamin C, E, B6, B complex, zinc, octacosanol, EFA (essential fatty acid), bee pollen, L-tyrosine, manganese, L-arginine, L-cysteine, selenium.

HERBS

Astragalus, red raspberry tea, damiana, Panax ginseng, sarsaparilla, saw palmetto, licorice root, unicorn root.

AROMATHERAPY

Jasmine, sage, patchouli, ylang ylang.

For infertility: The following script should be used in the morning and at night for at least six weeks. To optimize results, you may even want to try the scripts for in vitro fertilization, depression, stress, and general illness.

INFERTILITY SCRIPT

THE MAGIC MIRROR

Intention: To increase fertility.

Find a comfortable place where you won't be disturbed, and sit in a comfortable chair. Now sit back and relax with both feet on the floor, and place your hands on the armrests of the chair or in your lap — whichever is comfortable for you.

Concentrate as you breathe deeply, letting the air come into your nose and out your mouth. Concentrate and breathe IN with the nose and OUT with the mouth. IN with the nose and OUT with the mouth. And IN with the nose and OUT with the mouth. Now let's concentrate on breathing OUT with the mouth and IN with the nose. And OUT with the mouth and IN with the nose. And OUT with the mouth and IN with the mouth.

Imagine you are standing in front of a magic mirror. Look how pretty it is. As you look into the mirror, you can see how attractive you are. You notice your skin, your hair, your whole body and you feel very, very attractive. Look deeper into the mirror and see how fearless you are. You are filled with hope and your self-esteem feels so balanced. You see the beauty of who you are inside and out. This makes you very happy, relaxed, and stress-free. Feel how self-assured you are. How confident you feel.

(Close your eyes for a moment and feel what a beautiful person you are.)

As you look in the mirror, you magically see the insides of your body. When you look inside, you see everything in excellent working order. Look away from the image in the mirror and down at your body. Feel whatever it is that is inside your body that is stopping you from being healthy. Listen and hear your body tell you what it needs to be healthy and fertile. Listen. Listen. You may not hear the words but you know what you have to do to make your body like the one in the magic mirror. A body that is healthy, happy, and fertile.

(Close your eyes for a moment and listen to your body.)

Now feel your body shifting towards being healthy. Feel it shifting right now, in this time, in this place. Making your body healthy and whole. Making your body fertile and strong. You know what foods and nutrients you need, all the ones that are right for your body, and you want and crave only these right foods. Feel the shifting happening in your body. All your body's systems working properly and correctly. Feel the shift take place now.

(Close your eyes for a moment and feel the shift of your body.)

Look in the mirror and you see that your body is exactly like the one in the mirror. Healthy, strong, and fertile, and you feel such power.

Keeping this feeling with you, turn away from the mirror. Look to your left; there is a television set with a chair in front of it. Go over and sit down on the chair. The screen of the television is the most beautiful purple you have ever seen. Watch as this purple screen fades to white.

On the screen is a healthy human egg located in exactly the right place for successful fertilization. Watch as the sperm swim onto the screen. Watch as one of the virile healthy sperm makes its way into the egg.

(Close your eyes for a moment and watch the screen.)

The white light radiates off the screen and surrounds you. There is so much peace and happiness because you know you are becoming fertile. Everything in your body is shifting to perfection. Working correctly. You know and trust this.

(Close your eyes for a moment and feel the trust in your body and self.)

Feeling in control and filled with happiness and peace, walk back over to the magic mirror. Look at your image. It is perfect in every way. You are stress-free, without anxiety, peaceful, serene and happy, and you know these feelings will stay with you.

For in vitro fertilization, three scripts are given. Preparing the Garden should be used in the morning and at night prior to in vitro fertilization, Planting the Seed should be used during the in vitro fertilization process, and Growing the Flower should be used in the morning and right after implantation for as long as you need it. To optimize results, you may even want to try the scripts for infertility and stress.

IN VITRO FERTILIZATION SCRIPTS

PREPARING THE GARDEN
Intention: To increase fertility.

Find a comfortable place where you won't be disturbed, and sit in a comfortable chair. Now sit back and relax with both feet on the floor, and place your hands on the armrests of the chair or in your lap — whichever is comfortable for you.

Concentrate as you breathe deeply, letting the air come into your

nose and out your mouth. Concentrate and breathe IN with the nose and OUT with the mouth. IN with the nose and OUT with the mouth. And IN with the nose and OUT with the mouth. Now let's concentrate on breathing OUT with the mouth and IN with the nose. And OUT with the mouth and IN with the nose. And OUT with the mouth and IN with the mouth.

Imagine you are about to plant a wonderful garden and are standing in front of an area of earth. Look up to the sky, there are trees that are blocking the sunshine. Look down at the earth, it looks dry and hard.

Look to your left and you see all the tools you need to make your garden grow. These are two sets of golden tools — one large and one very, very small — and they glint in the sun. There may be a golden saw, a golden hoe, and golden bags of rich soil and fertilizer; whatever you need to make the earth fertile is right next to you. You know that the large tools are to make the garden fertile. You know that the tiny tools will go inside your body, making you fertile. You trust that as you use the large golden tools to prepare your garden, the tiny golden tools will automatically go into your body and prepare your body.

(Close your eyes for a moment and look at the golden tools.)

Watch as you pick up the golden tools you need to create your fertile garden. Watch as you use the tools to clear away all the debris and place the debris in the golden bags and haul them away from the garden. Watch as you cut the trees, making a pathway for the sunlight to your garden. Watch as you till the soil and add the fertilizer until it is rich and loamy and ready for planting. Do whatever you need to for the garden to be fertile.

(Close your eyes for a moment and watch as your garden becomes fertile.)

Now look up and see the sun shining down on your soil. It is so rich and fertile. You feel that your body is rich and fertile. Everything is in proper working order. Reach down and touch the soil in your garden. Feel the richness on your fingers. You know your body is rich and fertile. Exactly right for you. Exactly right for the seed. Feel the power of the earth rise up from the ground and go through you. Feel the power. You are happy, content and peaceful, and you know that these feelings will stay with you.

PLANTING THE SEED
Intention: For successful implantation.

Find a comfortable place where you won't be disturbed, and sit in a comfortable chair. Now sit back and relax with both feet on the floor, and place your hands on the armrests of the chair or in your lap — whichever is comfortable for you.

Concentrate as you breathe deeply, letting the air come into your nose and out your mouth. Concentrate and breathe IN with the nose and OUT with the mouth. IN with the nose and OUT with the mouth. And IN with the nose and OUT with the mouth. Now let's concentrate on breathing OUT with the mouth and IN with the nose. And OUT with the mouth and IN with the nose. And OUT with the mouth and IN with the mouth.

Imagine you are in your garden. This is the day to plant the seed and you are very excited, but relaxed and calm. You are happy because you know that your garden is going to grow the most beautiful flower that anyone has ever seen.

(Close your eyes for a moment and see this beautiful flower.)

To your right is a golden trowel and a small gold box. Pick up the gold box and trowel and place them on the rich, fertile soil. Look in the box. There are three or four magic seeds. They glint and sparkle in the sun. How wonderful these seeds are. You know that one of these seeds will produce your most beautiful flower.

(Close your eyes for a moment and look at the seeds.)

Look at the ground, it is so fertile. Look up at the sky. It is a clear, beautiful blue and the sun is shining warmly and brightly. Look to your left; there is a golden watering can filled with magic water. You know that everything is right for your seed to grow. You feel, know, and trust this. Everything is ready for your wonderful, magic seed. The seed that will grow into your beautiful flower that you want, desire, and need. Everything is ready and the time is finally here. You feel a deep sense of relaxation and peace enter into your body.

(Close your eyes for a moment and feel the relaxation and peace.)

Plant your seeds in your garden. There can be no mistake. Everything is right for you in this time, in this place, right now. Feel the relaxation, peace and joy.

(Close your eyes for a moment and feel the joy.)

The seed is planted. Feel how comfortable the seed is. Send the seed love and feel it respond, feeling warm and protected. As you send the seed love, feel how comfortable it is. The seed knows it is in the right place. Feel how ready your seed is to grow into that beautiful flower. Feel the love between you and the seed.

(Close your eyes for a moment and feel the love between you.)

There is no doubt that this seed will grow. Feel your connection to the seed. You feel so relaxed, so positive, so happy. You know that the seed is comfortable and starting to grow inside of you. You can feel the tiny roots start to come out of the seed. The roots are attaching it to the fertile ground. The movement is slow and steady and sure. You have X-ray vision and can see inside the earth. Look at the seed's roots implanting themselves into the ground. Feel the roots growing and attaching themselves.

(Close your eyes for a moment and feel the attachment.)

You know that your flower is growing. It is strong and safe. You feel the love and bonding between you. Everything is perfect. Feeling peaceful, happy, without doubt and feeling relaxed, you know these feelings will stay with you.

GROWING THE FLOWER
Intention: For successful growth.

Find a comfortable place where you won't be disturbed, and sit in a comfortable chair. Now sit back and relax with both feet on the floor, and place your hands on the armrests of the chair or in your lap — whichever is comfortable for you.

Concentrate as you breathe deeply, letting the air come into your nose and out your mouth. Concentrate and breathe IN with the nose and OUT with the mouth. IN with the nose and OUT with the mouth. And IN with the nose and OUT with the mouth. Now let's concentrate on breathing OUT with the mouth and IN with the nose. And OUT with the mouth and IN with the nose. And OUT with the mouth and IN with the mouth.

Imagine you are in your garden. The sun is shining and the sky is the most beautiful blue you have ever seen. The temperature is exactly right for you. You are so peaceful in your garden. All your stress, all your worry seems to melt away as you stand in your garden in the sunshine.

You have X-ray eyes. Look down into the earth and check on your seed. You see the seed's roots firmly implanted in the ground. You know that your flower is growing. Look at how the roots are getting all the nourishment they need from the soil. The roots are strong and healthy. Your seed is strong and healthy. You feel and know this.

(Close your eyes for a moment and feel how healthy the seed is.)

Now watch as you see the top of the flower pushing out of the ground. You know that whatever this flower needs to grow, it will receive without effort. Everything is so right. Raise your right or left hand, whichever is good for you. Look at the palm of your hand. You see a white light coming out of your palm's center. The light is nourishing, protective, nurturing, and healing. Watch as the rays of white light come out of the palm of your hand.

(Close your eyes for a moment and see the white light.)

Now place your hand over the flower and watch as the white light from your hand caresses the flower. See how the white light comforts your flower. You feel this white light is nurturing the flower and giving it strength. You know the flower is growing strong in this white light. Watch as the white light comes from your hand and goes into the flower, giving it strength. Helping it to grow. You know this is happening in this time, this place, right now.

(Close your eyes for a moment and feel the flower growing strong.)

Feel the flower taking whatever it needs from this wonderful white light. Feel the flower growing strong and getting everything it needs. The flower is growing up towards the sun, its roots steadfast in the rich, fertile earth. The flower is getting all the nourishment it needs to grow healthy and strong.

(Close your eyes for a moment and feel the growth of the flower.)

Watch as the white rays of light recede into the palm of your hand. You are happy, relaxed, and stress-free, knowing you can come into the garden at any time to nourish and protect the flower with the white light from your hand. You smile and look up at the sun. Feeling joyful and relaxed, you know these feelings will stay with you.

CHAPTER 28

Insomnia

Sleep is essential to life. Lack of sleep may impair judgment, cause personality changes, and reduce accuracy and speed in doing repetitive mental or physical tasks. Sleeplessness that is experienced repeatedly is known as insomnia.

Insomnia can be caused by physical disorders of the organs, muscle aches, hypoglycemia, breathing problems, indigestion, pain, grief, stress, anxiety, and depression. Certain drugs and medications can cause insomnia. Watch out for decongestants, high blood pressure medicine, antidepressants, and anti-seizure medications. Lack of copper, calcium, magnesium, and iron, and too much caffeine can contribute to insomnia and to a sleep cycle in which you wake up every few hours.

There are two types of sleep: REM (rapid eye movement) and NREM (non-REM). Most dreams occur during REM sleep in the dreamtime stage, in which the cerebral cortex is active, muscle activity is inhibited, breathing and heartbeat are irregular, and body temperature is less controlled. During NREM sleep, the cerebral cortex is less active, muscles can move, and fewer dreams are reported.

REM and NREM sleep alternate in cycles. Normally, REM sleep occurs about every 90 minutes. The amount of sleep required is dependent on age. Newborn babies spend two-thirds of their time sleeping. Young adults require one-third of their time for sleep, and older adults need less sleep, but go to bed and rise earlier.

There are certain recognized maladies that contribute to insomnia. In restless leg syndrome (RLS), people can't seem to keep their legs still. Legs may jerk, twitch, and kick involuntarily, or get muscle cramps. There may be a heredity factor in RLS. In circadian rhythm disorder, the internal body clock (circadian rhythm) is out of synch with the daily 24-hour clock. The circadian rhythm can be short or long in people with this disorder. People with a short circadian rhythm go to sleep early and are said to have "advanced sleep syndrome"; people with a long circadian rhythm go to bed later and are said to have "delayed sleep syndrome." SAD (seasonal affective disorder) is also a circadian rhythm disorder; it is linked to the shortage of sunlight during the winter months. In conditional insomnia, a person can't fall asleep anywhere except in his or her own bed. Sleep apnea is a condition of snoring and irregular breathing; breathing can actually stop for as long as two minutes during such sleep. This creates an oxygen deprivation in the blood, which generally awakens the sleeper.

Sleeping pills, over-the-counter sleep medications, and prescription drugs may interfere with REM sleep, enhance dependency, and worsen insomnia. They also may cause side effects of drowsiness, confusion, anxiety, restlessness, depression, dry mouth, and enlarged prostate.

To overcome insomnia, establish a daily routine prior to sleep, use your bed only for sleeping and intimate activity, try not to nap during the day, exercise in the late afternoon or early evening, take a hot bath, and try stress-reduction techniques like relaxing music, meditation, and self-hypnosis. Other natural therapies include acupuncture, aromatherapy, proper diet, and herbal therapies.

Insomnia Relief Remedies

MENTAL ATTITUDE
Cause: procrastination and attachment.
Cure: let go, live in the moment, take action.

FOODS & DIET
Avoid: alcohol, sugar, chocolate, soft drinks, caffeine, food colorings, additives, preservatives, processed meats, and processed foods.
Good Foods: watercress, lettuce, filberts, almonds, broccoli, chicken (dark meat), turkey, milk, peanuts, bananas, honey.

VITAMINS & SUPPLEMENTS
Multivitamin and mineral supplement with whole foods and enzymes, B complex, zinc, calcium, magnesium, inositol, melatonin.

HERBS
Cumin, California poppy, hops, wild lettuce, passion flower, valerian, chamomile.

AROMATHERAPY
Jasmine, sage, patchouli, ylang ylang.

The following scripts should be used in the morning and at night for at least six weeks. To optimize results, you may even want to try the scripts for anxiety and stress.

INSOMNIA SCRIPTS

RELAXATION
Intention: To eliminate insomnia.

Find a comfortable place where you won't be disturbed, and sit in a comfortable chair. Now sit back and relax with both feet on the floor, and place your hands on the armrests of the chair or in your lap — whichever is comfortable for you.

Concentrate as you breathe deeply, letting the air come into your nose and out your mouth. Concentrate and breathe IN with the nose and OUT with the mouth. IN with the nose and OUT with the mouth. And IN with the nose and OUT with the mouth. Now let's concentrate on breathing OUT with the mouth and IN with the nose. And OUT with the mouth and IN with the nose. And OUT with the mouth and IN with the mouth.

Imagine you are lying in bed. The bed is the most comfortable bed you have ever been in. The sheets are your favorite color, the pillows are exactly right for you. This is a magic bed. As you lie in the bed, you feel your body start to relax. You realize that this bed is gently rocking you back and forth. In such a gentle rhythm it rocks you back and forth. This rhythm is one that is right for you.

As you lie on the bed, you start to feel all the tension, all the stress start to flow out of your body.

(Close your eyes for a moment and feel how relaxed you are.)

Starting with the forehead, feel all the tension just melt away. Feel all the worry just melt away from your mind and body. Your eyes become heavy and your face begins to relax. A warm sensation enters into your head, making you feel so very, very calm. So very, very relaxed.

Feel the warmth go into your neck and shoulders now. Feel all the stress, all the tension just melt away as the comfortable bed rocks you gently back and forth. You are becoming more and more relaxed.

Now feel this warmth enter into your back and all your muscles in your back just begin to relax. The tension and stress just leave the back area as the warmth comes into the top of your back and radiates down the back ever so gently. Feel the stress and tension leaving your back area. Making you feel so peaceful, so calm, so relaxed.

Now feel the warmth enter into your buttocks and down the backs of your legs. Feel all the stress and tension leave these areas right now. The warmth permeates to the bottom of your feet and around each foot. Feel each and every toe just relax more and more as you become so calm, so stress-free. Without any tension in the whole back area of your body. Feeling so relaxed.

Now feel the warmth go up the abdominal area and into your chest and down your arms to each and every finger. Feel all the muscles, all the bones, all the nerves, all the tissues and every fiber of your being release any tension. Just becoming relaxed as all the tension and all the stress just melt away from your body, as you get deeper and deeper relaxed. So very, very relaxed. Without a care or worry in the world. You just feel a deep, deep sense of relaxation.

You are so calm. So centered. So relaxed, as the bed gently rocks back and forth and back and forth in such a gentle rhythm.

(Close your eyes for a moment and feel how relaxed you are.)

You feel so very relaxed. Your eyes are heavy. Your mind is relaxed. Your body is relaxed. You are more relaxed than you have ever been before and you know that this feeling will stay with you.

THE BUBBLE
Intention: To eliminate insomnia.

Find a comfortable place where you won't be disturbed, and sit in a comfortable chair. Now sit back and relax with both feet on the floor, and place your hands on the armrests of the chair or in your lap — whichever is comfortable for you.

Concentrate as you breathe deeply, letting the air come into your nose and out your mouth. Concentrate and breathe IN with the nose and OUT with the mouth. IN with the nose and OUT with the mouth. And IN with the nose and OUT with the mouth. Now let's concentrate on breathing OUT with the mouth and IN with the nose. And OUT with the mouth and IN with the nose. And OUT with the mouth and IN with the mouth.

Imagine yourself in a field of green grass. Flowers dot the field and their smell is so sweet. Exactly as you like them. It is sunset and the sky is filled with very soft beautiful colors. Clouds dot the sky and the sun's reflection shows the setting sun in all its splendor.

Look ahead of you to the far right; a forest of trees stands tall against the sky. As you look towards these trees you see something moving towards you. It is as if it is floating towards you. You feel safe and secure and know nothing can harm you here. Watch as the movement comes nearer. As it comes into view, you see that it is a very large transparent bubble. The bubble is etched in white light. As it approaches you the bubble becomes bigger and bigger.

(Close your eyes for a moment and look at the bubble coming towards you.)

The bubble is now floating very gently in front of you. It is bigger than you are. Watch as the bubble floats in front of you. Now lift up your hand and touch the bubble. Watch as your hand goes into the bubble. The bubble does not break. The bubble is still floating gently before you. You know that this bubble is a safe place. Step inside the bubble.

(Close your eyes for a moment and watch as you step inside the bubble.)

When you enter the bubble, everything is so peaceful and quiet. A gentle serenity comes into your body. All your thoughts, all your troubles, all your stress, all your tensions are left outside of the bubble. You start to feel very, very relaxed. You feel all the restlessness leave your body. In this bubble your body is working perfectly. Any physical symptoms you seem to have just disappear. You are breathing regularly and evenly. It is so peaceful and quiet here in this softly floating bubble. Your body clock is regulated and right for you. Feel the gentle shifting and changing as your mind and your body become quiet and relaxed.

(Close your eyes for a moment and feel how relaxed your body is.)

Now feel how your mind is relaxing. Any stress, any anxiety just melts away from your mind. You feel centered, relaxed, and peaceful. You begin to feel relaxed, happy, and whole. Self-empowered and able to handle anything in your life without stress, without tension. All negative feelings are just melting, melting away right now. Leaving your mind feeling more relaxed than you have ever known it to be.

(Close your eyes for a moment and feel how relaxed your mind is.)

You know you will be able to rest whenever and wherever you need to, without effort. Relaxation and rest will just happen. You trust in this and it becomes a part of you. Watch as the bubble starts to shrink around you. Watch and feel the bubble outlining your body. This bubble will stay with you. This outline makes you feel centered, calm, and relaxed, and you know that these feelings will stay with you.

CHAPTER 29

Low Self-Esteem

Self-esteem is shaped by a person's behavior and actions, as well as by society, culture, and important individuals throughout a person's life. Self-esteem is more than self-worth. It is a confidence in your own ability to think, to make decisions, to cope with life challenges, and to feel worthy of your success through happiness and enjoyment of your accomplishments. A basic need, self-esteem affects every area of life, including love and other relationships, and your work environment. True self-esteem manifests itself with realism, intuitiveness, flexibility, rationality, cooperation, and benevolence.

Symptoms of low self-esteem include feelings of inadequacy, guilt, shame, and inferiority, or a lack of self-trust, self-acceptance, and self-love. Low self-esteem plays a part in substance abuse, anxiety, depression, codependency, violent crimes, fear of intimacy, underachievement, sexual disorders, and aimlessness.

There are nine things that can help change low self-esteem:

1. Live consciously. Be aware of what you do and what effect it has on you and the world around you.

2. Practice self-acceptance. Accept the reality of your feelings, desires, dreams, wants, and needs without shame or resentment.

3. Let go of abnormal guilt.

4. Treat yourself with compassion and forgiveness.

5. Take responsibility. Accept that you, and only you, are responsible for your values, choices, dreams, actions, behavior, and personal happiness.

6. Honor yourself. Be self-assertive and honor your wants, needs, values, and their form of expression in truth and balance.

7. Live with purpose. Live productively by finding purpose, formulating goals, identifying and taking actions to achieve the goals, and monitoring these actions and outcomes to access achievement.

8. Maintain personal integrity. Integrate ideals, standards, and beliefs with your behavior. Do what you say and say what you do.

9. Be patient.

By taking an active part in your process, you will support and strengthen your self-esteem. There are several tools that you can use to raise self-esteem: humor, aromatherapy, Bach flower remedies, dreams, visualization, positive affirmations, and self-hypnosis.

Low Self-Esteem Relief Remedies

MENTAL ATTITUDE
Cause: fear of change.
Cure: positive thinking and action.

FOODS & DIET
Avoid: alcohol, sugar, caffeine, food colorings, additives, preservatives, processed meats, and other processed foods.
Good Foods: yogurt, oat bran, turnips, sardines.

VITAMINS & SUPPLEMENTS
Multivitamin and mineral supplement with whole foods and enzymes, B complex, Vitamin C, zinc, calcium, magnesium.

HERBS
Cumin, basil, coriander.

AROMATHERAPY
Jasmine, lavender, rose.

The following scripts should be used in the morning and at night for at least six weeks. To optimize results, you may even want to try the scripts for anxiety and stress.

LOW SELF-ESTEEM SCRIPTS

THE TIDE POOL
Intention: To increase self-esteem.

Find a comfortable place where you won't be disturbed, and sit in a comfortable chair. Now sit back and relax with both feet on the floor, and place your hands on the armrests of the chair or in your lap — whichever is comfortable for you.

Concentrate as you breathe deeply, letting the air come into your

nose and out your mouth. Concentrate and breathe IN with the nose and OUT with the mouth. IN with the nose and OUT with the mouth. And IN with the nose and OUT with the mouth. Now let's concentrate on breathing OUT with the mouth and IN with the nose. And OUT with the mouth and IN with the nose. And OUT with the mouth and IN with the mouth.

Imagine you are walking by the ocean. The sun is shining and glinting happily off the water. The sand is the most beautiful color you have ever seen. As you walk along the beach you notice a group of rocks. Walk over to the rocks and look down in between them. You see a tide pool there. The water is calm and clear. As the sun reflects into the water you see yourself reflected in the water.

As you look into the tide pool, it becomes like a mirror. You see yourself as you are meant to be. Full of confidence and able to make decisions. You feel the power in yourself as you look at your reflection in the tide pool.

(Close your eyes for a moment and feel how powerful you are.)

Touch the water and watch as the ripples you have created edge to the sides of the tide pool. Watch as the water becomes still again. Look into the tide pool and as you do you see yourself enjoying life, being happy, and accomplishing what you need to do without indecision. You feel good about what you are accomplishing. How very wonderful this feels!

(Close your eyes for a moment and feel how good you feel.)

Now look into the pool and see that there are many people around you. Look at the people and see how they accept you. Feel how you are beginning to accept yourself. Feel the love that emanates from you and direct this love to your image in the tide pool. You know you are taking care of yourself. You are doing what is right for you in truth and integrity. Feel the power of your self-love as it comes into your body, making you strong. You are a special person in your own right and you feel worthy. You know you are special. You feel this inside and outside your mind and body.

(Close your eyes for a moment and feel how special you are.)

Watch as you begin to treat yourself with respect. Feel how you can trust yourself. You know you can make the right decisions for you. Feel the confidence flood your body. Feel it grow as it invades your mind, making you strong and whole as you have never been before.

(Close your eyes for a moment and feel how confident you are.)

Place your hand in the tide pool and watch again as the ripples go throughout the pool and become still. Your image seems to be the middle of a flower. A beautiful flower with you at its center. Watch as your petals fall off one by one by one. Any guilt, any shame, any negative feeling that you have about yourself just drops away, just like the petals of the flower. One by one by one.

As each petal drops off, your image in the center of the flower becomes bigger, stronger. Watch the petals drop off and see how strong you are becoming. You feel in control, confident, centered, happy.

Now watch as the image in the tide pool merges with you. Filling you to the brim with confidence, joy, happiness. You are filled with self-trust and acceptance, and you know this feeling will stay with you.

THE CITY STREET
Intention: To increase self-esteem.

Find a comfortable place where you won't be disturbed, and sit in a comfortable chair. Now sit back and relax with both feet on the floor, and place your hands on the armrests of the chair or in your lap — whichever is comfortable for you.

Concentrate as you breathe deeply, letting the air come into your nose and out your mouth. Concentrate and breathe IN with the nose and OUT with the mouth. IN with the nose and OUT with the mouth. And IN with the nose and OUT with the mouth. Now let's concentrate on breathing OUT with the mouth and IN with the nose. And OUT with the mouth and IN with the nose. And OUT with the mouth and IN with the mouth.

Imagine you are in a city. The hustle and bustle of the traffic and people are all around you. Hear the horns. See the colors of the cars. The buildings around you are tall and there are many people walking on the streets. You are one of these people, walking slowly. You are aware of who you are and what you are doing. As you look at the people passing by, you realize that they are the same as you. They are different shapes, different sizes, but you see that their basic wants and needs are exactly the same as yours.

(Close your eyes for a moment and look at the people.)

As you watch each person, you realize that you can accept yourself as you truly are. Your feelings, desires, dreams are valid. You know this in the very core of your being. Feel the self-acceptance come through your body. It is warm and feels so good and reassuring. Feel the feeling of self-acceptance fill your body, and as it does any shame, any guilt, any resentment just melts away. You feel so confident.

(Close your eyes for a moment and feel your self-acceptance.)

Now look to your right; there is a store there. Look into the store window and see your reflection. Look at how wonderful you are; you are now able to forgive yourself because you know you can now treat yourself with the compassion and love you well deserve. This brings such a feeling of joy and contentment into you body, mind, and spirit.

(Close your eyes for a moment and feel the contentment.)

As you look in the store window at your reflection, you know that you are responsible for your happiness and your choices. You know you are the only one who is in control of them. Look into the window and stare deep into your eyes. Feel the trust you have in yourself expand inside your body and mind. Feel this feeling. This self-trust gives you happiness, joy, and power.

(Close your eyes for a moment and feel how powerful you are.)

Now feel how you honor yourself by being in balance. Living in truth and reality. Knowing you can accomplish anything you want. You have the power. You know you will take an active part in your life. Consciously making decisions that are right for you, taking the action to make your life full and happy.

Feel the power within you. The trust. The joy. The confidence. And you know these feelings will stay with you.

CHAPTER 30

Memory Loss

Memory is the process the brain uses to store and retrieve information. There are three types of memory: sensory memory or perception, short-term memory, and long-term memory. Sensory memory is associated with the five senses (e.g., the taste of honey, the color of the sky, the sound of drums). Sensory memories are stored in a long-term, relatively permanent sensory memory buffer in the brain. Short-term memory is associated with speech; it includes information that is used in a given moment (e.g., remembering a telephone number). Long-term memory is associated with the meaning of a situation and not just the retention of details (e.g., conversation with a loved one).

With all three types of memories, the brain encodes each one, places them into "programs" with other memories, and then interconnects them to the brain's network. The brain's programs and interconnections are altered every time a new memory is added. The brain also encodes your values, choices, dreams, actions, behavior, and personal happiness in the same way as the three types of memories.

Occasional memory lapses are normal and can occur at any age. As we age, the ability to remember does not deteriorate, and memory can be maintained well through 90 years of age.

Various things can cause memory loss. Some diseases, such as thyroid disorders, hypoglycemia, chronic fatigue syndrome, allergy, and *Candida,* can cause memory loss. Inside the brain, memory loss can occur because of poor blood circulation, insufficient neurotransmitters, or insufficient nutrients permeating the brain because of cholesterol and triglycerides in the blood. An electric current passing through the brain, a blow to the head, substance abuse, and nutritional deficiencies (e.g., lack of amino acids or B vitamins) also affect memory.

Many people associate memory loss with Alzheimer's disease, which is a common type of dementia. Alzheimer's is a progressive mental deterioration that impairs memory and abstract thought functions in the brain. However, this is only one of its symptoms. Disorientation in space and time; inability to concentrate or communicate; depression; loss of bowel and bladder function; mood swings; and personality changes are additional symptoms. Both memory retrieval and the creation of new memories are impaired. Insufficient nutrients, exposure to high levels of aluminum and mercury (e.g., from dental amalgams), and the immune system's attacking the brain cells may play key roles in the development of Alzheimer's. Other disorders that can cause dementia similar to Alzheimer's are: hardening of the arteries, syphilis, brain clots and tumors, and a series of minor strokes.

It is possible that aluminum plays a role in Alzheimer's. Aluminum can be absorbed into your system if you use aluminum cookware, or from food additives, buffered aspirin, certain dandruff shampoos, antacids, antidiarrhea medicine, and deodorants. Look at the labels to see if any form of aluminum is listed before purchase.

There are several natural health care methods to use to improve memory: acupuncture, aromatherapy, Bach flower remedies, homeopathy, vitamin and herbal therapies, and self-hypnosis.

Memory Loss Relief Remedies

MENTAL ATTITUDE
Cause: ignoring emotional facts in your environment.
Cure: live in the moment and release attachment.

FOODS & DIET
Avoid: alcohol, sugar, caffeine, food colorings, additives, preservatives, processed meats, and other processed foods.
Good Foods: guava, rose hips, parsley, grapefruit, cauliflower, mangoes, molasses, watercress, lentils, brazil nuts, coconut, banana, alfalfa, lamb, beef, broccoli, almonds, artichokes, eggs, vinegar, sardines, yogurt, oat bran, turnips, kelp.

VITAMINS & SUPPLEMENTS
Multivitamin and mineral supplement with whole foods and enzymes, selenium, SOD (superoxide desmutase), zinc, Vitamin C, E, boron, lecithin, inositol, amino acids, manganese, RNA, DNA.

HERBS
Ginkgo biloba, gotu kola, dill, sage, coriander, cumin, rosemary.

AROMATHERAPY
Basil, cardamom, peppermint, rosemary.

The following self-hypnosis scripts are not for dementia diseases, but for memory loss of other origin. They should be used in the morning and at night for at least six weeks.

MEMORY LOSS SCRIPTS

THE STARS
Intention: To improve memory.

Find a comfortable place where you won't be disturbed, and sit in a comfortable chair. Now sit back and relax with both feet on the floor, and place your hands on the armrests of the chair or in your lap — whichever is comfortable for you.

Concentrate as you breathe deeply, letting the air come into your nose and out your mouth. Concentrate and breathe IN with the nose and OUT with the mouth. IN with the nose and OUT with the mouth. And IN with the nose and OUT with the mouth. Now let's concentrate on breathing OUT with the mouth and IN with the nose. And OUT with the mouth and IN with the nose. And OUT with the mouth and IN with the mouth.

Imagine you are floating in the night sky. The sky is dark around you. There are many sparkling stars. Look at how the starshine throws light into the dark sky. How very beautiful it is. You have a bag with you. You are going to collect five of the most beautiful stars and place them in your bag. As you float in the night sky, look at all the stars and select five of them that are just right for you and place them in your bag.

(Close your eyes for a moment and collect the stars.)

Now close the top of the bag and feel how your body is gently floating back down to the earth. You land in a room which is painted your favorite color. You feel very safe in this room. Open up your bag and take out a star. Hold the star in your open palm and watch as the star starts to move towards the ceiling. Feel the star's light come into your mind. You know that this starlight is improving your short-term memory. Ever so gently, feel the starlight shifting and changing your mind to whatever is right for you to improve your short-term memory. As your short-term memory improves, watch as the star by the ceiling fades and disappears. Your mind is absorbing the magic starlight to improve your short-term memory.

(Close your eyes for a moment and feel your short-term memory improve.)

Take out another star from your bag. Watch as it moves to the ceiling. Feel the star's light start to enter into your mind. You know that this starlight is improving your long-term memory. Feel the shifting, the changing in your mind as the starlight improves your long-term memory. Watch and see your mind absorbing the starlight as the star by the ceiling starts to fade away.

(Close your eyes for a moment and feel your long-term memory improving.)

Take out the third star. This starlight improves your perception. This starlight seems brighter as it enters your mind. Feel your mind absorbing the starlight, taking whatever it needs to improve your perception. Feel this light go to all of your five senses. Feel the healing, shifting, changing of these senses. Your eyes, your ears, your touch, your smell, your taste are all improving as your perception improves. Feel your perception becoming sharp. Watch and see this star by the ceiling fade and disappear as your mind and all five senses absorb what they need to improve your perception.

(Close your eyes for a moment and feel your perception improving.)

Take out the fourth star. This star can heal your body. Feel the star's light enter into your body as it moves up towards the ceiling. You feel the light shining bright and true as it enters into your body. This light corrects anything in your body that is stopping you from having a clear, good, sharp memory. Feel the starlight balancing your body. Making your body healthy and whole. The starlight is giving you everything you need. Watch as the star fades away, leaving you relaxed, healthy, and healed.

(Close your eyes for a moment and feel your body healing.)

Take out the fifth star. This is the brightest star of them all. It is the star of positive attitude. Feel this starlight enter into whatever part of your mind and body that it needs to. Feel the light shine, making you positive, joyful, and happy. Making you aware of what's going on. Turning anything negative into a positive. How wonderful this feeling is.

(Close your eyes for a moment and feel how positive you are.)

Now hold out your hand and watch the star come back into your palm. This powerful star can fit into your pocket. As you place this star in your pocket you know that you can use this star anytime you need to.

You feel happy, healthy. You know your memory has improved, and this feeling will stay with you.

UNIVERSAL LIGHT
Intention: To improve memory.

Find a comfortable place where you won't be disturbed, and sit in a comfortable chair. Now sit back and relax with both feet on the floor, and place your hands on the armrests of the chair or in your lap — whichever is comfortable for you.

Concentrate as you breathe deeply, letting the air come into your nose and out your mouth. Concentrate and breathe IN with the nose and OUT with the mouth. IN with the nose and OUT with the mouth. And IN with the nose and OUT with the mouth. Now let's concentrate on breathing OUT with the mouth and IN with the nose. And OUT with the mouth and IN with the nose. And OUT with the mouth and IN with the mouth.

Imagine you are sitting in a secluded glade. There is a brook running behind you and the water is gently babbling. You feel quite relaxed and safe sitting among the trees. As you look up you see a patch of blue sky. Every once in a while a cloud slowly floats by. It is so peaceful here sitting and relaxing in this glade.

(Close your eyes for a moment and feel how relaxed you are.)

As you sit, feeling so relaxed, you can see a golden light come from out of the sky. It is the most unusual light but it seems so peaceful. Watch as the light forms into a steady beam that points to the top of your head. Feel it attach to the top of your head and you feel a gentle, soothing warmth enter into you. It is as if this golden beam of light attaches you to the sky and even beyond.

(Close your eyes for a moment and feel the warmth of the light.)

As the light enters into your mind, you feel peaceful and know that the light contains all the knowledge, all the power to improve your memory. Feel the light speed the circulation to the brain to whatever it is that is right for you to improve your memory. Feel how the light balances the body, giving it all the information it needs to support, improve, and retain your memory. You know that your mind and your body are shifting and changing to improve your memory.

(Close your eyes for a moment and feel the changes taking place.)

Stay attached to this universal golden light as long as you need to. When you are done, watch the golden light recede back into the sky. You feel changed and happy, filled with information. Your memory is sharp and clear and you know that this will stay with you.

CHAPTER 31

Menopause

Menopause is a natural part of life. It is the point when a woman stops ovulating and menstruating, and fertility ends. During this time, ovary production of the hormones estrogen and progesterone stops. The other endocrine glands take over and begin producing some of the estrogen and other hormones that the body needs at this time.

Estrogen is necessary not only in reproduction; it contributes to normal cell function in the arteries, brain, bladder, bones, breasts, heart, liver, skin, and vagina. Complicated chemical interactions produce three types of estrogen: estrine (E1), estradiol (E2), and estriol (E3).

Menopause is an individualized process for each woman. Symptoms vary in the types experienced, their length, and time. The average age for the start of menopause is 51 years and 3 months; menopause can last up to five years. Peri-menopause, or pre-menopause, may begin as a very slow process around the age of 35 and will continue until actual menopause occurs.

Some of the symptoms of menopause are: hot flashes, dizziness, emotional symptoms (e.g., mood swings, anxiety, depression), numbness in the arms, heart palpitations, insomnia, night sweats, headaches, vaginal dryness and infection, low libido, urinary tract infections and incontinence, and heavy or irregular menstrual periods. Osteoporosis is not a symptom of menopause, but it is associated because of the decrease in estrogen levels, which may affect cellular bone growth.

Hormone replacement therapy (HRT), estrogen replacement therapy (ERT), and natural replacement therapy (NRT) are available. HRT and ERT have side effects and may increase the risk of breast and ovarian cancer, and the autoimmune disease lupus. Synthetic estrogens are laboratory made and accumulate in the body. They can cause changes in the liver, high blood pressure, fluid retention, and blood clots. Other estrogens used in ERT are from equine (horse) estrogen, which is extracted from pregnant mare's urine. This type of estrogen, which is considered a natural estrogen, may cause changes in the liver and may have other risks. Also found in this type of ERT is a type of horse estrogen called equiline, which humans do not have in their bodies. Selection of HRT or ERT requires researching the facts about the side effects and long-term effects prior to choosing which therapy is right for you.

Phytoestrogens, a form of natural replacement therapy, are plant-based compounds that mimic estrogen in the body and do not have any known side effects. In fact, phytoestrogens work even more gently than human estrogen in the body. Plant estrogens are found in soybeans, black beans, fava beans, red kidney beans, and other beans, and in herbs.

Plant estrogen contains isoflavones. Isoflavones are composed of two substances: daidzein and genistein. These substances fall into the molecular niches that normal human estrogen settles into. Isoflavones can help perimenopausal women with endometriosis, uterine fibroids, and abnormal tissue growth.

Diet plays a major role in managing menopause. Exercise is just as important and helps to reduce the risk of osteoporosis. Sex is important during menopause, because it helps decrease symptoms of vaginal dryness and helps hormonal balance. Having a positive attitude is the best thing you can do for treatment of menopause. Positive emotions boost the mind, body, and spirit, which helps in minimizing and eliminating symptoms.

There are many natural health care methods that are of help during menopause: diet, acupuncture, aromatherapy, Bach flower remedies, homeopathy, vitamins, supplements, herbal therapies, visualization, yoga, tai-chi, and self-hypnosis.

Menopause Relief Remedies

MENTAL ATTITUDE
Cause: reluctance to adjust to change.
Cure: practice receiving and giving.

FOODS & DIET
Avoid: alcohol, sugar, dairy products, caffeine, food colorings, additives, preservatives, processed meats, and other processed foods.
Good Foods: low-fat, high-fiber, mostly vegetarian diet; broccoli; legumes including beans, soybeans, yellow lentils, black-eyed peas; sunflower seeds; flaxseed oil; garlic; filberts; watercress.

VITAMINS & SUPPLEMENTS
Multivitamin and mineral supplement with whole foods and enzymes; Vitamin C, E, B12, B complex, niacin; bioflavonoids, calcium, magnesium, boron, silica, manganese.

HERBS
Basil, dill, evening primrose oil, wood betony, dong quai, vitex, black and blue cohosh, wild Mexican yam, red clover, ginseng, ginkgo biloba, St. John's wort, yellow dock, stinging nettle, cranberry, marshmallow root, uva ursi, vervain, motherwort, false unicorn root, licorice root, coriander, cumin.

AROMATHERAPY
Geranium, rose, sage, chamomile, cypress, fennel, jasmine, neroli, eucalyptus, lavender, ylang ylang.

The following scripts should be used in the morning and at night for at least six weeks. To optimize results, you may even want to try the scripts for aging, stress, anxiety, depression, memory loss, general illness, headaches, osteoporosis, pain, and vertigo.

MENOPAUSE SCRIPTS

THE CAKE
Intention: To eliminate physical symptoms of menopause.

Find a comfortable place where you won't be disturbed, and sit in a comfortable chair. Now sit back and relax with both feet on the floor, and place your hands on the armrests of the chair or in your lap — whichever is comfortable for you.

Concentrate as you breathe deeply, letting the air come into your nose and out your mouth. Concentrate and breathe IN with the nose and OUT with the mouth. IN with the nose and OUT with the mouth. And IN with the nose and OUT with the mouth. Now let's concentrate on breathing OUT with the mouth and IN with the nose. And OUT with the mouth and IN with the nose. And OUT with the mouth and IN with the mouth.

Imagine you are in the most beautiful kitchen you have ever seen. The sunlight is coming in through the windows. Everything is so light and airy and the smells in this kitchen are so wonderful. This kitchen has every type of convenience, every utensil you might ever need.

This is a magic kitchen and the cabinets are filled with every kind of ingredient. Even if you don't like to cook or don't know how you feel, you would like to cook in this magic kitchen. You know that anything you make will require very little effort and will come out perfect every time. You can't make a mistake.

(Close your eyes for a moment and see this beautiful kitchen.)

You are going to make a magic cake. A magic cake without calories. A wonderful cake that will balance all your body's needs. Filled with all the ingredients in just the right amounts to provide exactly the right amounts of hormones and estrogen that you need. Go to the cabinet and open the door. Take out a bowl. Go to the cupboard and start pulling out ingredients. You don't have to know what they are, just pull out anything that feels or looks or smells right for you.

(Close your eyes for a moment and collect the ingredients.)

You may not know what some of them are, but you trust they are the right ones for you. These ingredients may balance your adrenal glands, your cholesterol, your DHEA and any other substances your body may need to stop irregular periods. Heavy periods. Pick out and measure the ingredients and place them in the bowl. These are the ingredients that are exactly right for your body. Place them in the bowl and blend them together. You are very happy knowing that this magic cake will automatically help you, without worry, without effort.

(Close your eyes for a moment and feel how happy you are.)

Now take out a cake pan and place the mixture into the pan. Put the pan in the oven. Watch the cake through the glass door. The cake rises and since this is a magic oven, the cake is cooked immediately. Take this wonderful magic cake out of the oven and let it cool for a few seconds. It smells so good! Go to the cabinet and take out a plate, a knife and a fork. Go back to the now cooled cake and cut yourself a piece that is right for you. Place it on the plate. Take it to the table and sit down. Pick up the fork and put a morsel of your magic cake into your mouth. Feel it disappear on your tongue. It is the most wonderful-tasting food you have ever had. Now feel how the cake is interacting in your body, giving your body everything it needs.

(Close your eyes for a moment and feel your body shifting.)

Eat as much cake as your body needs. Feel the shifting and changing in your body until it is exactly right and comfortable for you.

You feel balanced. Centered. Regular. Your body working at top efficiency. You smile and know you have accomplished much today. You know you will keep this feeling with you.

THE ROLLER COASTER
Intention: To eliminate emotional symptoms of menopause.

Find a comfortable place where you won't be disturbed, and sit in a comfortable chair. Now sit back and relax with both feet on the floor, and place your hands on the armrests of the chair or in your lap — whichever is comfortable for you.

Concentrate as you breathe deeply, letting the air come into your nose and out of your mouth. Concentrate and breathe IN with the nose and OUT with the mouth. IN with the nose and OUT with the mouth. And IN with the nose and OUT with the mouth. Now let's concentrate on breathing OUT with the mouth and IN with the nose. And OUT with the mouth and IN with the nose. And OUT with the mouth and IN with the mouth.

Imagine you are on a roller coaster. Going up and up and up and then coming down very, very fast. Up and down. You go over small heights and then big heights. Rhythmically going up and down very, very fast. Feel the air around you. Hear the whoosh of the ride. Up and down. Up and down.

(Close your eyes for a moment and feel the roller coaster.)

Now watch as the roller coaster starts to slow down and comes to very flat ground. It starts to go slower and slower. It is going slowly now, down a very straight level path at a speed that is comfortable for you. You look in front of you and see a beautiful blue tunnel ahead. Beautiful blue lights are coming out of the tunnel.

You start to feel peaceful and know that you are safe. You have nothing to fear. Watch as the roller coaster enters into this beautiful blue tunnel. The inside of the tunnel is lined with beautiful blue crystal. The lights bouncing off the blue crystal walls seem to glimmer and shine. Making beautiful patterns all around you. It is so beautiful. You feel so peaceful. So safe. So secure. What beautiful peaceful lights. You've never felt so relaxed. In fact you are more relaxed than you have ever known yourself to be.

(Close your eyes for a moment and feel how relaxed you are.)

You feel this beautiful crystal blue light go into your body and your mind. Making you feel centered. Making you happy as you feel this wonderful blue light absorbing all the depression, all the negativity, all the irritability that you may have. Absorbing it away from your body. Away from your mind. Balancing you. Balancing your moods. Making you calm and peaceful.

(Close your eyes for a moment and feel how balanced you are.)

Now watch and feel how the blue light makes your memory sharp and clear. Feel how sharp your memory is. Feel how the blue light is balancing your hormones. Making the levels exactly right for you. Making you calm, centered, peaceful. Feel the power swell within you as you become a woman of knowledge and wisdom. Notice how good you feel. This feeling will stay with you.

(Close your eyes for a moment and feel how good you feel.)

Now watch and feel how the crystal blue light goes to any place that you have stress or tension or pain. Feel the light absorbing them away. Each and every one. Watch and feel as the blue light comes out of your body, taking with it any negativity, stress, pain and tension. Leaving you feeling so centered. In control. Peaceful. Happy.

(Close your eyes for a moment and feel how centered you are.)

Now feel the roller coaster start to move slowly out of the tunnel. It comes to a stop. Get out of the roller coaster and look up at the beautiful blue sky. Feel how balanced and centered you are. How happy and peaceful you are. How powerful you are. This feeling will stay with you.

THE BREATH
Intention: To eliminate hot flashes.

Find a comfortable place where you won't be disturbed, and sit in a comfortable chair. Now sit back and relax with both feet on the floor, and place your hands on the armrests of the chair or in your lap — whichever is comfortable for you.

Concentrate as you breathe deeply, letting the air come into your nose and out your mouth. Concentrate and breathe IN with the nose and OUT with the mouth. IN with the nose and OUT with the mouth.

And IN with the nose and OUT with the mouth. Now let's concentrate on breathing OUT with the mouth and IN with the nose. And OUT with the mouth and IN with the nose. And OUT with the mouth and IN with the mouth.

Imagine that each breath you inhale is absorbing the heat in your body. With each exhalation out of your mouth, the breath takes the heat out of your body. Inhale, absorbing the heat. Exhale, releasing the heat.

Watch and feel the breath and how it goes into the body, finding the heat in your face, your neck. Watch as the breath absorbs the heat, making you feel cooler, more centered. Exhaling the breath as the heat is leaving your body. Continuing breathing deeply. Absorbing the heat and letting it out of your body, breath by breath. Getting centered. Feeling cooler. Feeling very, very calm. Feel how much cooler you are.

Watch and feel the heat leave your body. You feel relaxed, cool, and in control, and you know this feeling will stay with you.

CHAPTER 32

Obesity

Obesity is an excess of body fat. It is caused by a combination of physical, emotional, nutritional, and environmental stress. Some of the factors that contribute to weight gain are physical, like illness, glandular malfunction, slow metabolism, and lack of exercise. There can be emotional factors like eating for the wrong reasons, holding onto weight for control, and food dependency. Nutritional factors could include poor diet, improper amounts of food, poor absorption of nutrients, and an impaired digestive process. Pollutants and toxins from environmental sources can come from internal sources (for example, drugs that have side effects of weight gain) or external sources like smog, which weakens the immune system and slows down the body's food processing system. An individual's weight gain or loss is always a unique process. The combination of factors contributing to weight gain and retention are as varied as each person.

Obesity can crowd the space of internal organs, and place stress on the joints, back, and legs. It also increases a person's susceptibility to infection, diabetes, liver damage, heart disease, high blood pressure, kidney disease, stroke, and gall bladder disease.

There are seven steps to successful weight loss: 1) make a total commitment, 2) decrease emotional stress, 3) change your eating habits, 4) get exercise, 5) release stress and stay motivated, 6) keep positive, and 7) learn to think thin with self-hypnosis. Remember: "You are what you think" is just as important as "You are what you eat."

Eight keys can be used with self-hypnosis to maximize weight loss:

*Choose the right foods. Try a low-fat, high-fiber mostly vegetarian diet.

* Don't skip meals. Eat smaller, more frequent meals throughout the day.

* Drink water. At least 1 gallon of water daily.

* Avoid toxins, especially drugs, caffeine, and alcohol.

* Use fat-burning vitamins, minerals, supplements, and herbs.

* Exercise. Build lean muscle tissue by exercising at least three times a week for 30 minutes.

* Be supportive of yourself. Treat yourself kindly and set realistic goals.

* Get adequate sleep.

Diuretic herbs, lipotropic vitamins, and natural appetite suppressants can help, but a commitment and change to a healthier lifestyle can bring permanent weight loss.

Meals of balanced proteins, complex carbohydrates, and some fats can help balance blood sugar and burn fat more effectively. Eat the right kinds of fat that contain essential fatty acids and eliminate saturated fats from your diet. Avoid crash diets to reduce the risk of heart disease.

Natural remedies include a proper diet, aromatherapy, acupuncture, homeopathy, herbal, vitamin, and supplement therapy, relaxation methods, visualization, and self-hypnosis.

Obesity Relief Remedies

MENTAL ATTITUDE
Cause: fear of hurt.
Cure: trust yourself. Use positive thought and take action. Learn to receive as well as give.

FOODS & DIET
Avoid: alcohol, nicotine, caffeine, dairy foods, salt, sugar, white flour, white rice, sodas, fried foods, food colorings, additives, preservatives, processed meats, other processed foods.
Good Foods: low-fat, high-fiber, mostly vegetarian diet; whole grains, legumes, artichokes, asparagus, lentils, turkey, tuna, swordfish, halibut, shark, chicken, watermelon, cantaloupe, pineapple, squash, turnips, parsley, avocados, lemon, almonds, radishes, corn, celery, cucumbers, spinach, grapefruit, strawberries, kale, lettuce, onions, apples, barley and wheatgrass juice, apples, rice cakes, yogurt, popcorn, flaxseed oil.

VITAMINS & SUPPLEMENTS
Multivitamin and mineral supplement with whole foods and enzymes, Vitamin C, bioflavonoids, L-arginine, L-lysine, GABA (gamma-aminobutyric acid), L-ornithine, choline, inositol, coenzyme Q10, zinc, acidophilus, betaine hydrochloric acid, L-carnitine, lecithin, chromium picolinate, kelp, L-glutamine, L-tyrosine, chitosan.

HERBS
Alfalfa, peppermint, basil, fennel, uva ursi, dandelion, parsley, garcinia cambogia, ginger, cayenne, clover, astragalus, aloe vera, corn silk, horsetail, hyssop, oat straw, juniper berries, thyme, yarrow, cardamom, cinnamon, licorice root, fenugreek, ginseng.

AROMATHERAPY
Fennel, juniper, patchouli.

The following scripts should be used in the morning and at night for at least six weeks. To optimize results, you may even want to try the scripts for low self-esteem, guilt, anxiety, energy, and stress.

OBESITY SCRIPTS

THE MAGIC WALL
Intention: To eliminate excess weight.

Find a comfortable place where you won't be disturbed, and sit in a comfortable chair. Now sit back and relax with both feet on the floor, and place your hands on the armrests of the chair or in your lap — whichever is comfortable for you.

Concentrate as you breathe deeply, letting the air come into your nose and out your mouth. Concentrate and breathe IN with the nose and OUT with the mouth. IN with the nose and OUT with the mouth. And IN with the nose and OUT with the mouth. Now let's concentrate on breathing OUT with the mouth and IN with the nose. And OUT with the mouth and IN with the nose. And OUT with the mouth and IN with the mouth.

Imagine you are in a house. It is the most beautiful house you have ever seen. The colors of the carpets are your favorite colors. Everything is perfect in this house. There is a staircase going up to another level. Walk up the stairs. With each step that you take, you feel more and more relaxed. Go up the stairs until you reach the next level of the house.

(Close your eyes for a moment and feel how relaxed you are.)

When you reach the next level, there is a very long hallway. Go down the hallway and enter the first room that you see at your right. Inside the room is a long white wall. Go over to the wall and watch it turn into a mirror. Touch the glass of this mirror. You feel safe and calm. Step into the mirror. As you reach the other side of the mirror, turn around and look back at it. Your reflection is exactly as you would like to be. You are at your correct weight. Your clothes fit so well. You are happy and healthy with your body at exactly the right weight for you.

(Close your eyes for a moment and see yourself at your perfect weight.)

As you look in the mirror, you feel your mind start to change. You are so positive and you know you will lose weight. You will be this person in the mirror. Feel the commitment enter into your body. Feel the motivation as it seeps into your mind. You know that the commitment and motivation are strong. You feel this with every fiber of your being.

(Close your eyes for a moment and feel the commitment and motivation.)

Look in the mirror and feel how your mind is shifting, making you thin. In your mind you are positive. You know that the emotions that have tied you to eating will no longer affect you. You will not desire to eat when you have negative feelings. Whenever a negative feeling happens, a positive one will take its place. Watch and feel all your feelings turning into positive ones that are right for you. Feel yourself releasing any of your emotional ties to eating right now.

(Close your eyes for a moment and feel how positive you are.)

Now watch as your mind releases all the negative behavior patterns that are stopping you from losing the weight you want and need to lose. Feel your mind shifting, changing, releasing these patterns one by one.

(Close your eyes for a moment and feel the release of negative eating patterns.)

Watch as the mirror shows you sitting down at a table and eating. The table has all the foods that are right for you. Watch yourself eat these right foods. They taste so good and these are the foods that you desire. This is the type of food you need and want. You no longer desire any food that is not good for you. Whenever you see a food that is not good for you, the desire just melts away. It just disappears, leaving you wanting only the foods that are right for you.

(Close your eyes for a moment and see yourself eating the right foods.)

Watch yourself eating the right foods. Eating exactly the right amounts of food. You have no desire to overeat. When you are full, you no longer want any extra food. You see yourself chewing slowly, enjoying your food. See yourself eating your food slowly. You have no desire to overeat, it just melts away. Feel how satisfied you are without overeating. Feel this happening now.

(Close your eyes for a moment and see yourself eating the right amount of food.)

Watch as the mirror shifts, showing you exercising in the mirror. No matter what you are watching, it is right for you. Feel your fat turn into lean muscle tissue as you exercise. Watch the fat turn into muscle. You like to exercise because you know that every time that you do, you are losing weight. Your body is strong, healthy. Look at your body, perfect in every way. You are motivated to exercise. Feel this feeling come over you. See how healthy your mind and body are in the mirror, just exercising.

(Close your eyes for a moment and see yourself happily exercising.)

Look at your image in the mirror. You are so healthy and fit. All of your body's systems are in perfect working order. You know you are committed and motivated. Look at yourself at your perfect weight. See how your clothes fit. You are sleek and strong. You want to eat the right foods. You have no desire to overeat. You feel so positive. Step through the mirror and back to the other side. Turn around and look into the mirror. You feel full of motivation, energy, and happiness. You know you are losing weight right now. These feelings will stay with you.

WEIGHT-LOSS MAGIC
Intention: To lose weight.

Find a comfortable place where you won't be disturbed, and sit in a comfortable chair. Now sit back and relax with both feet on the floor, and place your hands on the armrests of the chair or in your lap — whichever is comfortable for you.

Concentrate as you breathe deeply, letting the air come into your nose and out your mouth. Concentrate and breathe IN with the nose and OUT with the mouth. IN with the nose and OUT with the mouth. And IN with the nose and OUT with the mouth. Now let's concentrate on breathing OUT with the mouth and IN with the nose. And OUT with the mouth and IN with the nose. And OUT with the mouth and IN with the mouth.

Imagine you are in a kitchen. It is so comfortable here. You feel relaxed and safe. On the counter there is a bottle of pills. The label says MAGIC PILLS. Open the bottle and take one out. Place the pill in the palm of your hand. The pill is all natural, safe, and has no side effects. The pill is such a pretty color. Pour a glass of water and take the pill. Feel the pill go into your body. Your appetite is decreasing. Feel the magic pill breaking down in your body. It is absorbing all the fat out of your body. Feel the fat become attracted to the pill bits and being absorbed. Feel the excess fluid in your body being absorbed. All the excess fat and as much excess water as is right for you is being absorbed by the pill.

(Close your eyes for a moment and feel the fat and water being absorbed.)

You know that this magic pill has decreased your appetite and absorbed the excess water and fat out of your system. Now look at the counter. There is a bottle of liquid there. This is a special formula that is all natural and safe. It cannot hurt you. Get a glass of water and place a tablespoon of this magic liquid in the water. Stir this mixture and look at the tiny sparkling lights within the glass. Drink the liquid down. It has a very pleasant taste. Feel the liquid enter into your body. Feel your body responding by increasing your metabolism. Your digestive system is shifting to perfect working order. Feel the energy in your body. Your body is boosting itself to perfect working order.

(Close your eyes for a moment and feel your perfect body working.)

Feel your collagen production increase to the right amount for you. Look at your skin — see how wonderful it looks. This is promoting your weight loss, taking away all your aches and pains. Feel your energy and stamina increase as the fat in your body turns into lean muscle tissue. Feel and watch the lights in your body shifting, changing you until your body is in perfect working order.

(Close your eyes for a moment and feel your perfect body.)

You feel filled with energy, positive, committed, motivated and happy, and you know that these feelings will stay with you.

CHAPTER 33

Osteoporosis

Osteoporosis is excessive bone porosity or tissue reduction caused by loss of minerals in the bone substance. It is a progressive disease that causes weakness in the bones and bone structure, which makes bone fractures more likely to happen. Women are more likely to have osteoporosis than men are.

Bone tissue is the body's storage area for calcium, which is used in the blood, nerves, and many other body tissues. In normal adults, bone is continually being made and replaced. Many factors are necessary for this to occur, including enough dietary calcium and phosphorus, and vitamins A, C, and D. Several hormones also are involved in bone growth. Bone consists of fibers of collagen, which provide elasticity, and calcium and phosphorus, which give hardness. In osteoporosis, the thinning is mainly due to the loss of collagen, which takes the calcium with it. In osteoporosis, the new bone growth does not keep up with the absorption of old bone; the result is thinning of the interior bone mass, and actual spaces in the bone.

Primary osteoporosis, also called senile or post-menopause osteoporosis, is the most common. There are two types of primary osteoporosis: Type I and Type II. Type I is caused by hormonal changes like loss of estrogen and Type II is caused by a dietary deficiency of calcium and vitamin D, and to a lesser degree boron, copper, zinc, silicon and manganese. These dietary deficiencies result in decreased absorption of calcium in the bone. Dairy foods may contribute to osteoporosis and do not provide enough calcium for the body.

Risk factors that influence osteoporosis include small body frame; the larger and denser the bone, the less chance of osteoporosis. Race is a factor: Northern European and Asian women are more likely to develop osteoporosis than African women are. Other risk factors are: family history; anorexia; poor diet; lack of exercise; substance abuse; smoking; excessive caffeine; liver, kidney, endocrine, and thyroid disease; and long-term use of corticosteroids, antiseizure medications, and anticoagulants.

Symptoms of osteoporosis usually go unnoticed. They can manifest themselves as general aches and pains, compression fractures, nerve and organ crowding, loss of height, tooth loss, back pain, and susceptibility to fractures.

Secondary osteoporosis is also called disease osteoporosis, and comes from bones that have been immobilized by paralysis, traumatic fractures, or prolonged weightlessness like space flight.

The best way to handle osteoporosis is to prevent it. There are several natural health care methods that help people with osteoporosis: a low-fat, mostly vegetarian diet; acupuncture; aromatherapy; homeopathy; vitamin, supplement, and herbal therapies; yoga; tai-chi; and self-hypnosis.

Osteoporosis Relief Remedies

MENTAL ATTITUDE
Cause: feeling too old to learn or change.
Cure: be flexible and build new goals.

FOODS & DIET
Avoid: alcohol, sugar, carbonated drinks, animal fats, caffeine, food colorings, additives, preservatives, processed meats, and other processed foods.
Good Foods: low-fat, high-fiber, mostly vegetarian diet; broccoli, sesame seeds, nuts, sunflower seeds, berries, corn, soybeans, molasses, wheat germ, liver, watercress, carrots, rose hips, kale, red peppers, swordfish, egg yolks, caviar, bananas, spinach, tuna, salmon, lentils, almond milk, yogurt.

VITAMINS & SUPPLEMENTS
Multivitamin and mineral supplement with whole foods and enzymes, Vitamin A, C, E, D, K, beta carotene, selenium, boron, calcium, magnesium, folic acid, manganese, phosphorus, glucosamine sulfate, copper, zinc, L-lysine, L-arginine.

HERBS
Black cohosh, oat straw, nettle, feverfew, ginseng, alfalfa, barley grass, dandelion, garlic, parsley, cumin.

AROMATHERAPY
Rose, lavender, sage, eucalyptus.

The following scripts should be used in the morning and at night for at least six weeks. To optimize results, you may even want to try the scripts for pain.

OSTEOPOROSIS SCRIPTS

THE SPA
Intention: To eliminate osteoporosis.

Find a comfortable place where you won't be disturbed, and sit in a comfortable chair. Now sit back and relax with both feet on the floor, and place your hands on the armrests of the chair or in your lap — whichever is comfortable for you.

Concentrate as you breathe deeply, letting the air come into your nose and out your mouth. Concentrate and breathe IN with the nose and OUT with the mouth. IN with the nose and OUT with the mouth. And IN with the nose and OUT with the mouth. Now let's concentrate on breathing OUT with the mouth and IN with the nose. And OUT with the mouth and IN with the nose. And OUT with the mouth and IN with the mouth.

Imagine you are in a spa. You are completely alone and peaceful. To your left, you see a whirlpool bath. It looks so relaxing. Smell the aromatic oils in the air as you start to feel the tension coming out of your body. The whirlpool is exactly the right temperature for you. Sit down in the whirlpool and watch as the soft bubbling water turns into multicolored lights. The lights are bubbling around you softly. You feel so comforted watching these beautiful swirling, bubbling multicolored lights.

(Close your eyes for a moment and feel how relaxed you are.)

Feel the lights go into your body. The emerald green light. The electric blue light. The ruby red light. The brilliant yellow light, going gently into your body. Making you feel safe, calm, centered. Feel the lights going around your bones inside your body. Surrounding your bones. Penetrating softly, gently into your bones. It feels so good.

(Close your eyes for a moment and feel how good you feel.)

Feel the lights enter your joints and your cartilage. Ever so gently. Without pain. Just softly surrounding and entering your skeletal structure all over your body. You feel so relaxed, more relaxed than you have ever known yourself to be. These lights are filled with calcium and other nutrients that your bones, your joints, your cartilage may need to make them strong. Feel the lights building up your bones, your joints, your cartilage. Giving them everything they need to make them strong. Building up the bone density. Increasing the bone density wherever there is a loss. You feel this. You know this. You trust that this is happening right now, in this time, in this place.

(Close your eyes for a moment and feel your strong, dense bones.)

The lights are making you strong. Balancing your body. Feel the multicolored lights working. You are so calm and peaceful. So relaxed. You are healing your bones. You feel this happening. Your bones feel strong. Your body chemistry is working properly. Your joints are supple. Whatever you need, you are getting right now!

Feel the strength. Feel the power. Now step out of the whirlpool. Feel the energy, the peacefulness. Feel the strength. You feel wonderful and you know your bones are stronger. Denser. You are feeling very happy and healthy. You know this feeling will stay with you.

THE TREE
Intention: To eliminate osteoporosis.

Find a comfortable place where you won't be disturbed, and sit in a comfortable chair. Now sit back and relax with both feet on the floor, and place your hands on the armrests of the chair or in your lap — whichever is comfortable for you.

Concentrate as you breathe deeply, letting the air come into your nose and out your mouth. Concentrate and breathe IN with the nose and OUT with the mouth. IN with the nose and OUT with the mouth. And IN with the nose and OUT with the mouth. Now let's concentrate on breathing OUT with the mouth and IN with the nose. And OUT with the mouth and IN with the nose. And OUT with the mouth and IN with the mouth.

Imagine that you are in a backyard. The sky is blue and cloudless. There is an old oak tree in the yard. It is very big and stately. There are a lot of branches on this tree and they spread out over the yard.

You have X-ray vision and can see into the tree. Looking at the branches, you find that some of the branches are weak. These branches do not have much substance or density inside them. The tree seems bent over in the wrong places.

(Close your eyes for a moment and look at the tree.)

To your right you see a shed. Go over to the shed and look inside. There are large bags of nutrients, hormones, and other things that the tree could use to make it strong. Look to your left and in the shed you see a bucket. Take out the bucket and mix some of the nutrients from the bags in it. You seem to know exactly what the tree needs and can make no mistakes. Mix the nutrients together.

(Close your eyes for a moment and mix these healing nutrients together.)

Walk over to the tree. Spread the nutrients all around the base of the tree. There is a garden hose behind you. Pick up the hose and turn on the water. Water the nutrients at the base of the tree. When you are done, put the hose away and look at the tree. With your X-ray eyes, you can see the nutrients being absorbed into the tree. Look and feel how the tree is getting stronger. See all the nutrients go to every branch, every twig of the tree. The branches are getting stronger. The twigs are getting stronger. The tree looks straighter.

(Close your eyes for a moment and see the tree getting stronger.)

As you watch the tree getting stronger, you feel your own nutrients becoming balanced and your own bones getting stronger. Watch the tree absorb the nutrients; feel your bones growing denser, stronger. You feel your own bones becoming uncompressed. You feel your aches, pains, and back pain disappearing. Watch the tree. Feel your body. How strong you feel. As the tree becomes straighter, so do you. Feeling your bones getting stronger and denser.

(Close your eyes for a moment and feel your bones.)

Now look at the tree. See how steadfast and tall it is. How healthy it is. The branches gently rustle in the breeze almost as if to say "thank you." You feel your own body strong and healthy. Your bones feel strong and dense. You are happy and know you have done good work today. You know this feeling will stay with you.

CHAPTER 34

Pain

Pain can be agonizing. It is an unpleasant sensory and emotional experience usually associated with strenuous activity, disease, or injury of body tissue. It can also be caused by toxins within the body systems. Pain is the body's warning system. It is the messenger that brings information about a problem that is happening within the mind and body.

The nervous system has sense organs called nociceptors that are found in muscles, organs, skin, blood vessels, and other structures in the body. These sense organs convert stimulation from injuries into impulses that are transmitted up the spinal cord to the brain centers. When an injury occurs, the spinal reflexes are activated, which causes the muscles to spasm around the injury. The spasms protect the injury by minimizing blood loss. These spasms also produce a cramping pain, which stimulates the release of substances that cause inflammation and pain.

There are three types of pain: low-level, acute, and chronic. Low-level pain motivates you to rest the injured area so repair can take place. Acute pain needs immediate attention, and chronic pain is continual, intermittent, or cyclical pain that never seems to disappear, even after healing of the injury.

Pain is a two-step procedure. The first step is the physical reality of the pain. The second step is how you process the pain. After the reality of the pain is felt, people will process it differently. People may feel anxious, tense, discouraged, helpless, or become hypochondriacs. They may even overuse prescription drugs. These types of actions lead to holding on to the pain, which inhibits the healing process. A positive attitude can help boost the immune system, which may help to eliminate the pain faster. Sometimes, desensitizing the painful areas for a short time can alleviate the pain.

There are many natural ways to help eliminate chronic pain, including: acupuncture; acupressure; biofeedback; chiropractic care; cold and heat therapy; diet and lifestyle changes; herbal therapy; homeopathy; massage therapy; magnet therapy; vitamin, mineral, and supplement therapy; meditation; visualization; and self-hypnosis.

Pain Relief Remedies

MENTAL ATTITUDE

Cause: refusal to accept learning.
Cure: be aware of what you are doing and live in the moment.

FOODS & DIET

Avoid: alcohol, sugar, carbonated drinks, caffeine, food colorings, additives, preservatives, processed meats, and other processed foods.
Good Foods: low-fat, high-fiber diet, pineapple, garlic, papaya, saffron, radishes, barley.

VITAMINS & SUPPLEMENTS

Multivitamin and mineral supplement with whole foods and enzymes, Vitamin C, E, B6, B2, MSM (methylsulfonylmethane), GLA (gamma linoleic acid), papain, trypsin, L-carnitine, glucosamine sulfate, magnesium, calcium, phenylalanine.

HERBS

Aloe vera, catnip, licorice root, angelica, willow bark, rosemary, kava, hops, cayenne pepper, chamomile, ginseng, wood betony, parsley.

AROMATHERAPY

Juniper, lavender, rosemary.

The following scripts should be used in the morning and at night for at least six weeks. To optimize results, you may even want to try the scripts for arthritis.

PAIN SCRIPTS

THE SPIRAL STAIRCASE

Intention: To eliminate pain.

Find a comfortable place where you won't be disturbed, and sit in a comfortable chair. Now sit back and relax with both feet on the floor, and place your hands on the armrests of the chair or in your lap — whichever is comfortable for you.

Concentrate as you breathe deeply, letting the air come into your nose and out your mouth. Concentrate and breathe IN with the nose and OUT with the mouth. IN with the nose and OUT with the mouth.

And IN with the nose and OUT with the mouth. Now let's concentrate on breathing OUT with the mouth and IN with the nose. And OUT with the mouth and IN with the nose. And OUT with the mouth and IN with the mouth.

Imagine you are in a hallway of a very old house. You are standing in the entryway, and there is a spiral staircase at the center of the hall. Look at the faded rug going up the stairs. Grab the handrail and start walking up the stairs. As you ascend the spiral staircase, you feel yourself going higher and higher. You keep going 'round and 'round on the spiral staircase. Level by level, step by step.

(Close your eyes for a moment and see yourself climbing the spiral staircase.)

Stop at the level that is right for you. You see an old door there. The old door is locked, but you see a golden key in the keyhole. Turn the key and walk into the room. The room is large and airy with many windows. It is a very comfortable room. On the wall in the room is a very large mirror. Walk over to the mirror and stand before it.

As you look at your image in the mirror, you see red areas wherever you have pain in your body. The red areas may be inside or outside your body, but you see them all.

(Close your eyes for a moment and see the red painful areas.)

Tell your image in the mirror that you are in pain. Ask the image in the mirror to find the cause of the pain and eliminate it for you. You trust your image in the mirror because you know it is your higher self and it can do anything. Your mirrored image understands what you need and why you need it. Watch as your image smiles at you. You start to feel very, very relaxed.

(Close your eyes for a moment and feel how relaxed you are.)

Watch in the mirror as healing white light starts to surround your body. Watch as this white light goes around to every red pain spot inside and outside your body. Feel the white light absorbed into each area of pain. Feel the soothing and healing of each pain spot taking place in this time, right now. Feeling the healing taking place and how each pain is slowly disappearing, one by one by one. Feel the healing taking place in your body.

(Close your eyes for a moment and feel the white light healing the pain.)

All the pain is disappearing from your body. Watch as the white light absorbs all the red, painful areas, leaving you pain-free. Now watch as the white light slowly disappears, taking with it any remnants of the pain that is left. As the light disappears all your pain is gone.

Smile at your image in the mirror and thank it for the help it has given you. Watch as your mirrored image smiles back. Turn away from the mirror, walk through the door, and close it. Lock the door with the golden key and place the key in your pocket. This is your special place that you can come to at any time to alleviate your pain. Turn around and walk down the spiral staircase. With each step you feel how pain-free and happy you are, and you know this feeling will stay with you.

THE SAND DUNE
Intention: To eliminate pain.

Find a comfortable place where you won't be disturbed, and sit in a comfortable chair. Now sit back and relax with both feet on the floor, and place your hands on the armrests of the chair or in your lap — whichever is comfortable for you.

Concentrate as you breathe deeply, letting the air come into your nose and out your mouth. Concentrate and breathe IN with the nose and OUT with the mouth. IN with the nose and OUT with the mouth. And IN with the nose and OUT with the mouth. Now let's concentrate on breathing OUT with the mouth and IN with the nose. And OUT with the mouth and IN with the nose. And OUT with the mouth and IN with the mouth.

Imagine you are at a secluded beach. The sun is shining and the sky is a pretty blue. The ocean is lapping its waves onto the shore. Hear the seagulls cry overhead. Watch the waves as they roll in to the shore. It is so peaceful here. There are palm trees that sway gently in the breeze and the temperature is exactly right for you.

(Close your eyes for a moment and feel how peaceful you are.)

Look over to the right; there is a large, white sand dune. Walk over and sit on the sand dune, facing the ocean. As you sit down, the weight of your body seems to sink into the sand. Lie down on your back in the white sand. It is soft and feels so wonderful. Feel the sand as it starts to cover any part of your body that is in pain. Softly, gently covering that part of your body that is in pain. It is cool under this white sand. How good this sand feels on your body.

(Close your eyes for a moment and feel the sand on your body.)

Now feel the sand go inside your body and wherever there is a painful spot, feel the white sand start absorbing the pain away. All the aches, all the pain being absorbed into the sand and away from your body.

(Close your eyes for a moment and feel the sand absorbing your pain.)

You start to feel very good as each pain just seeps into the sand and away from your body. Watch as the sand goes into each and every pain spot in your body and absorbs the pain away. Do this for as long as you need, until every pain in your body is absorbed.

(Close your eyes for a moment and feel the sand absorbing your pain.)

Now watch and feel the sand coming out of your body the same way it went in. Feel how the sand is taking out your pain with it, out and away from your body. Each and every pain leaving you. You are pain-free and feel so good. You are happy and know that these feelings will stay with you.

CHAPTER 35

PMS

Premenstrual syndrome (PMS) is a name for a wide variety of physical, emotional, and psychological symptoms that occur a week or two prior to a menstrual period.

PMS begins in early puberty and is most common in women over 25 years of age. Although 75% of women experience PMS symptoms at some time in their lives, only 5% of women are incapacitated completely by PMS.

The symptoms can include one or more of the following: acne, water retention, bloating, headaches, backaches, cramps, breast swelling, breast tenderness, muscle aches, constipation, insomnia, mood swings, lethargy, depression, weight gain, irritability, hostility, clumsiness, fatigue, increased appetite, and food cravings.

PMS is a physical problem brought on by diet, stress, overall mental and physical health, hormonal imbalance, and fluctuation of estrogen and progesterone levels in the body.

In the three weeks of the menstrual cycle before menstruation, estrogen and progesterone levels are high and stimulate the production of beta-endorphin, which elevates mood and decreases pain. Just before menstruation, the estrogen and progesterone levels in the body decline, which drops the beta-endorphin level. When this level drops, insomnia, fatigue, irritability, and anxiety may occur. Prostaglandin levels, which regulate muscle contraction and inflammation, increase prior to and during menstruation. This may be responsible for pain, stress, and cramps. Mood swings and hostility may be related to the fluctuating levels of estrogen and progesterone and the lack of adequate calcium and magnesium in the body. Toxins found in dairy products, red meat, fried foods, food preservatives, caffeine and food additives may contribute to menstrual cramps.

There are four types of PMS, which are related to different symptoms:

PMS-A: anxiety, nervous tension, insomnia, mood swings.

PMS-B (also called PMS-H, for "hyperhydration"): water retention, salt retention, weight gain, bloating, breast swelling and tenderness.

PMS-C: cravings for sweets, low blood sugar, increased appetite, fatigue, headaches.

PMS-D: depression, withdrawal, lethargy, confusion, forgetfulness.

Doctors often prescribe ibuprofen or other drugs for PMS. There are side effects of taking these drugs every month that need to be researched before a decision is made to take them.

Natural methods of treating PMS include: acupuncture, Bach flower remedies, diet and lifestyle changes, exercise, herbal therapy, homeopathy, vitamin, mineral, and supplement therapy, meditation, visualization, and self-hypnosis.

PMS Relief Remedies

MENTAL ATTITUDE
Cause: insecurity or misuse of feminine energy.
Cure: learn to listen, be receptive and develop openness.

FOODS & DIET
Avoid: alcohol, sugar, salt, garlic, onions, raw salads, white potatoes, carbonated drinks, caffeine, food colorings, additives, preservatives, processed meats and other processed foods, hot spicy foods.
Good Foods: low-fat, high-fiber mostly vegetarian diet; salmon, tuna, mackerel, grains, flaxseed oil, evening primrose oil, royal jelly, molasses, wheat germ, kelp, watercress, parsley, artichokes, broccoli, soy, oats, peas, avocados, brown rice, sunflower seeds, almonds.

VITAMINS & SUPPLEMENTS
Multivitamin and mineral supplement with whole foods and enzymes, bee pollen, calcium, magnesium, zinc, Vitamin A, C, E, D, B6, B complex, bioflavonoids, lecithin, chromium picolinate, L-tyrosine, GLA (gamma linoleic acid), EPA (eicosapentaenoic acid).

HERBS
Angelica, dill, basil, lady's mantle, black cohosh, black haw, shepherd's purse, dandelion, cumin, blue cohosh, dong quai, red raspberry, vitex.

AROMATHERAPY
Sage, fennel, peppermint, rose, cypress, jasmine.

The following scripts should be used in the morning and at night for at least six weeks. To optimize results, you may even want to try the scripts for depression, general illness, pain, and stress.

PMS SCRIPTS

THE FLOWER GARDEN
Intention: To eliminate the emotional symptoms of PMS.

Find a comfortable place where you won't be disturbed, and sit in a comfortable chair. Now sit back and relax with both feet on the floor, and place your hands on the armrests of the chair or in your lap — whichever is comfortable for you.

Concentrate as you breathe deeply, letting the air come into your nose and out your mouth. Concentrate and breathe IN with the nose and OUT with the mouth. IN with the nose and OUT with the mouth. And IN with the nose and OUT with the mouth. Now let's concentrate on breathing OUT with the mouth and IN with the nose. And OUT with the mouth and IN with the nose. And OUT with the mouth and IN with the mouth.

Imagine you are in a flower garden. The colors are astounding. All of your favorite flowers are in the garden. There are even some types of flowers you have never seen. The smells are exotic and the riot of color is so pleasing to your eyes. Everywhere you look there are flowers. How beautiful it is here.

(Close your eyes for a moment and see the beautiful flowers.)

As you stand in the garden feeling so relaxed, you start to distinguish the different smells. Smell the lavender, the jasmine, and the rose scents as they tantalize your nostrils. Reach down and pick out a flower that you like. Breathe in the scent of the flower. As you breathe in and exhale the flower's scent, all the anxiety, the stress seems to go out of your body with each exhalation of your breath. Continue breathing in and out deeply, and feel how the tension is leaving your body and your mind. Keep breathing slowly and rhythmically.

(Close your eyes for a moment and feel the tension and stress leaving your body.)

Look down to your left and see a most unusual flower. It is the most beautiful flower you have ever seen. Reach down and pick the flower. See how beautiful each and every petal is. Bring the flower up to your nose and breathe in the smell. As the smell enters your nose, you feel your body balancing. Continue to breathe in the smell of the flower, and as you do, your body becomes calm and centered. You feel so balanced. Everything is quiet in your mind. You are so relaxed and centered.

(Close your eyes for a moment and feel how centered you are.)

As you continue to breathe in this pleasant flower scent, you feel all your irritability, all your stress, all your tension, all your anxiety just melt away. Feel a wonderful sense of warmth, joy, and happiness enter into your mind and body, making you whole and healthy right now. You know that this feeling will stay with you.

THE HERB SHOP
Intention: To eliminate the physical symptoms of PMS.

Find a comfortable place where you won't be disturbed, and sit in a comfortable chair. Now sit back and relax with both feet on the floor, and place your hands on the armrests of the chair or in your lap — whichever is comfortable for you.

Concentrate as you breathe deeply, letting the air come into your nose and out your mouth. Concentrate and breathe IN with the nose and OUT with the mouth. IN with the nose and OUT with the mouth. And IN with the nose and OUT with the mouth. Now let's concentrate on breathing OUT with the mouth and IN with the nose. And OUT with the mouth and IN with the nose. And OUT with the mouth and IN with the mouth.

Imagine you are in a very old herb shop. The smells are wonderful. There are herbs all around you. Some of the herbs are in pretty glass jars on the many shelves that are throughout the room. Some of the herbs are on tables and hanging from the ceiling. Everywhere you look there are herbs.

(Close your eyes for a moment and see all the herbs.)

In the middle of the room there is a large table. On the table is a green candle and a very old, antique book edged in gold and silver. There is a chair by the table. Walk over to the table, pull up the chair and sit down. There are matches by the candle. Pick one up, strike the match, and light the candle. The candle gives out the most beautiful green light you have ever seen.

Look at the book. It is very beautiful and old. You know it contains all the information on everything you need to do to heal your physical symptoms. Run your fingers over the cover. The book feels soft to your touch. Open the book and turn to any page. This page has all the information on the herbs that you need to heal. You cannot make a mistake. You may not see the words clearly on the page, but you know that your mind is absorbing all the information that you need to heal.

(Close your eyes for a moment and get all the information you need.)

Now close the book and look to your right. There is a large bowl. Pick up the bowl and go around the room and gather whatever herbs that you need to heal. Gather all the herbs that are right for you and place them in the bowl. The amounts and kinds of herbs that you take are exactly right for you and there can be no mistakes.

When you are done with your selection, go back to the table. There is a teapot there filled with boiling water. Open the lid of the teapot and place the herbs in the hot water. Put the lid back on and wait for the herbs to steep into a tea.

(Close your eyes for a moment and place the herbs in the teapot.)

Look at the candle shining its wonderful green light. Watch as the green light seems to come all around you. To your left there is a very beautiful teacup. The tea is ready; pour the tea into this cup. Drink the tea as you sit in the glow of this wonderful green healing light.

Feel how the tea is balancing your hormones, taking away all of your physical symptoms. Feel the green light of the candle go into your body, boosting the power of the herbs to heal you. The green light is making the herbs powerful and able to heal all the symptoms in your body without effort. Feel the healing taking place right now. Every tissue, every fiber, every organ, every bone in your body is being healed.

(Close your eyes for a moment and feel the healing taking place.)

You feel so wonderful, without any pain. You feel balanced and whole throughout your entire body. What a wonderful place this is — and you know you can come back here at any time. You smile and feel content, and you know this feeling will stay with you.

CHAPTER 36

Skin Diseases

The skin consists of the epidermis and the dermis. The surface of the skin consists of dead cells which have lost their internal structure and nuclei. As the dead skin is shed, it is replaced by the cells below. The epidermis is a thin layer of cells located below the dead cells and above the dermis. The epidermis gets its nutrition from the capillaries found in the dermis. The dermis is a fibrous mass that contains structures such as collagen fibers, elastic fibers, blood vessels, hair follicles, glands, lymphatic structures, and nerve endings.

The skin is the largest organ of the body. It protects the body, regulates body temperature, sensory perception, and immune response. The skin protects the body from invasion of bacteria, fungi, viruses, parasites, ultraviolet radiation, and mechanical injury. The body's temperature is regulated by the skin through the constriction and dilation of the dermal blood vessels around sweat glands, and it maintains heat through its insulating fat layer. Five sensory perceptions arise from the stimulation of the skin nerves: heat, cold, pressure, pain, and touch.

The skin responds when the immune system is attacked by releasing substances such as histamines and prostaglandins. These substances stimulate the nerve endings, which then cause pain, inflammation, redness, warmth, and swelling.

Skin diseases include tumors, physically and chemically caused disorders, and skin infections.

Physical and chemical agents can result in skin diseases when contact with the skin is made. These injurious agents include allergens, sunlight, ultraviolet light, heat, electricity, radiation, chemicals, pressure, and friction. These skin irritants can produce lesions, dermatitis, sunburn, poison ivy, bunions, corns, calluses, and heat rash. Some of the symptoms associated with these maladies include burning, itching, blistering, crusting, and pain.

Infectious skin diseases can be caused by bacterial, fungal, parasitic, and viral agents. Bacterial infections can include hair follicle infections such as folliculitis, furuncles, or boils. They are caused when bacteria enter into a break in the skin. Bacterial infections include a contagious disease known as impetigo. Fungal infections can include ringworm, which can occur on the scalp, body, or groin (where it is known as jock itch), or on the feet (athlete's foot). Fungus infection causes seepage of fluid, itching, stinging, and burning. Parasitic infections include scabies, caused by itch mites, which burrow into the skin and excrete waste products that cause intense itching, and lice, which can infect the scalp, body, or pubic area.

Viral infections of the skin include warts, herpes simplex virus (fever or cold sores), or herpes zoster (shingles). Shingles is caused by the same virus that causes chicken pox (*Herpes zoster*), which affects the nerve endings of the skin and can appear on any part of the body. Both non-cancerous and cancerous tumors (carcinomas) also can occur on the skin.

Acne is a skin disease which is more common in males. During puberty, hormonal changes to the endocrine glands can cause overactive oil glands in the skin. This excess oil traps bacteria in the pores. The exact cause of acne is unknown, but certain factors can contribute: oily skin, heredity, stress, allergy, drug use (e.g., lithium, oral contraceptives, steroids), nutritional deficiencies, junk food, menstruation, and chemical pollutants.

Natural methods of treatment include: acupuncture, diet and lifestyle changes, herbal therapy, homeopathy, vitamin, mineral, and supplement therapy, visualization, and self-hypnosis.

Skin Disease Relief Remedies

MENTAL ATTITUDE
Cause: insecurity of self.
Cure: communicate thoughts and ideas.

FOODS & DIET
Avoid: alcohol, tobacco, dairy products, sugar, caffeine, carbonated drinks, chocolate, food colorings, additives, preservatives, processed meats, and other processed foods.
Good Foods: low-fat, high-fiber, mostly vegetarian diet; almonds, apricots, pumpkin, squash, sweet potatoes, olive oil, sesame oil, horseradish, vinegar, watercress, avocado, cantaloupe, peas, lamb, eggs, broccoli, molasses, brewers yeast, wheat germ, yogurt, kelp, turkey, chicken.

VITAMINS & SUPPLEMENTS
Multivitamin and mineral supplement with whole foods and enzymes, Vitamin A, E, C, D, B12, B complex, zinc, L-cysteine, chromium picolinate, coenzyme Q10, selenium, beta carotene, bioflavonoids, grape seed extract, acidophilus, taurine, choline, folic acid.

HERBS

Burdock root, evening primrose oil, nettle, heartsease, garlic, oregano, aloe vera, red clover, yellow dock, figwort, tea tree, astragalus, bilberry, cayenne, alfalfa, dandelion root, rose hips, ginkgo biloba, pau d'arco, green tea, marshmallow root, oat straw, horsetail.

AROMATHERAPY

Chamomile, tea tree, rose, geranium, lavender, benzoin, juniper, sandalwood, myrrh, bergamot.

The following scripts should be used in the morning and at night for at least six weeks. To optimize results, you may even want to try the scripts for general illness and stress.

SKIN DISEASE SCRIPTS

THE WATERFALL
Intention: To eliminate skin problems.

Find a comfortable place where you won't be disturbed, and sit in a comfortable chair. Now sit back and relax with both feet on the floor, and place your hands on the armrests of the chair or in your lap — whichever is comfortable for you.

Concentrate as you breathe deeply, letting the air come into your nose and out your mouth. Concentrate and breathe IN with the nose and OUT with the mouth. IN with the nose and OUT with the mouth. And IN with the nose and OUT with the mouth. Now let's concentrate on breathing OUT with the mouth and IN with the nose. And OUT with the mouth and IN with the nose. And OUT with the mouth and IN with the mouth.

Imagine you are in a forest. It is hot outside and the sun is shining through the trees, making patterns on the ground before you. Listen to the birds chirping in the trees. You are walking along a dirt path that winds through the trees. As you make a turn in the path you see a waterfall. The water is glistening in the sun.

(Close your eyes for a moment and see the waterfall.)

You are alone and this is your private place where no one can enter. Take off your clothes and place them on a large rock that is to your right. Wade in the water and go over to the waterfall. The temperature of the water is exactly right for you. Go under the waterfall and feel how the water gently caresses your skin and your body. This is healing water, feel how it soothes your skin. It makes your skin feel so good.

(Close your eyes for a moment and feel how good your skin feels.)

Wherever the water touches your skin, you feel the healing taking place. Lift up your arms and feel how gently the water cascades around you. Feel your skin healing. The water is soothing your skin, taking away all the pain, the itchiness. How wonderful this feels. Feel the water healing your skin.

(Close your eyes for a moment and feel the healing taking place.)

You know that your skin is healing. You can feel it. Wade out of the waterfall and over to the side of the pool.

Look at your skin in the water. See how your skin has healed. Feel how your skin is whole and healthy. Feel the energy of your skin as it is being regenerated in this time, in this place right now.

(Close your eyes for a moment and see how your skin has healed.)

Walk out of the pool and over to the rock which has your clothes. You feel the sun's rays on your body drying you off. Hold your arms and hands up to the sun. Look at your skin — it is whole and healthy. Now put on your clothes. You smile and are happy, knowing your skin has healed. This feeling will stay with you.

THE DOCTOR'S OFFICE
Intention: To eliminate skin problems.

Find a comfortable place where you won't be disturbed, and sit in a comfortable chair. Now sit back and relax with both feet on the floor, and place your hands on the armrests of the chair or in your lap — whichever is comfortable for you.

Concentrate as you breathe deeply, letting the air come into your nose and out your mouth. Concentrate and breathe IN with the nose and OUT with the mouth. IN with the nose and OUT with the mouth. And IN with the nose and OUT with the mouth. Now let's concentrate on breathing OUT with the mouth and IN with the nose. And OUT with the mouth and IN with the nose. And OUT with the mouth and IN with the mouth.

Imagine you are in a doctor's office. Everything is sterile and clean. In the office there is an examination table and a chair. Take off your clothes, place them on the chair, and lie down on your back on the examination table. Look up to the ceiling and see a strange machine there. You are very relaxed and no one can enter the room. Look at the machine and you know that this machine can heal you. There is a switch beside the examination table; turn the switch on. Your favorite music starts to play and you become even more and more relaxed.

(Close your eyes for a moment and feel how relaxed you are.)

You hear a hum as the machine over your head switches on. The machine is sending magic air all over your body. The temperature is exactly right for you. Feel the magic air softly surround your skin. You feel the air surround your body and enter into all the layers of your skin. Your skin tingles pleasantly as the air enters into your body. Now feel how any bacteria, infection or virus just disappears as this soothing, wonderful air hits your body. Feel the air healing your skin right now. Feel how the skin is rejuvenating itself. The skin becoming so healthy.

(Close your eyes for a moment and feel your skin healing.)

When you are ready, turn over and lie on your stomach. The gentle air surrounds your skin. Feel how the air goes into each and every layer of your skin. Feel the air absorb all the impurities, all the pain, all the inflammation. The air is so soothing, so healing. Feel your skin healing.

(Close your eyes for a moment and feel your skin healing.)

When you are done, turn the switch to OFF. Get up off the table and walk over to the door. There is a full-length mirror there. Look at your skin in the mirror. See how your skin has healed. Look how healthy it looks. The skin is radiant. You feel happy and filled with energy and you know this feeling will stay with you.

THE MASK
Intention: To eliminate acne.

Find a comfortable place where you won't be disturbed, and sit in a comfortable chair. Now sit back and relax with both feet on the floor, and place your hands on the armrests of the chair or in your lap — whichever is comfortable for you.

Concentrate as you breathe deeply, letting the air come into your nose and out your mouth. Concentrate and breathe IN with the nose and OUT with the mouth. IN with the nose and OUT with the mouth. And IN with the nose and OUT with the mouth. Now let's concentrate on breathing OUT with the mouth and IN with the nose. And OUT with the mouth and IN with the nose. And OUT with the mouth and IN with the mouth.

Imagine you are in an old museum. It is so beautiful here, exactly as you pictured it would be. Look at the paintings, the color of the walls, the rugs. Everything seems balanced and warm. You are so relaxed here. Go over to the hallway and go into the first room you see. On the wall there are many masks. There is also an antique mirror in the corner of the room. Look at yourself in the mirror. Look at the masks on the wall. As you look at the masks you realize that there is one that has the exact features of your own face. The skin on the mask is free from blemish, free from acne. Look at how smooth the skin looks on the mask. Look at how you are meant to be.

(Close your eyes for a moment and look at the mask.)

Take the mask down from the wall and place it over your face. Look into the mirror. As you look into the mirror, you feel your own skin tingling beneath the mask.

Feel how this soft, gentle tingle seems to enter into your skin. You feel your skin changing beneath the mask. It is becoming healthy. Feel how your skin is healing.

(Close your eyes for a moment and feel your skin healing.)

Now feel how the soft, gentle tingle goes into your body. You know that this sensation is healing anything that is causing your problem. Feel the tingle balance your hormone levels to one that is exactly right for you. Feel the tingle adjusting all the systems of your body and destroying any bacteria. Feel the tingle making you healthy and whole right now, in this time, in this place.

(Close your eyes and feel your body healing.)

Now feel the tingle come out of your body the same way it went in. As this tingle goes out of your body, you know that it is healing any problem that is left in your body. Take off the mask and look in the mirror. Your skin is vibrant, radiant, and healthy. Your face is exactly like the mask and you know that it will stay that way. Your skin is whole and perfect in every way. You smile and feel happy and you know this feeling will stay with you.

CHAPTER 37

Stress

Every action or reaction comes from stress. Some stress is good because it motivates us to grow. Too much stress can cause emotional break-downs, fatigue, headaches, irritability, teeth grinding, high blood pressure, nervous twitches, sleep disorders, and even premature death. In fact, stress contributes to all mental and physical illness and disease.

The early warning signs of too much stress can show themselves on five levels:

* Physical level: pain, illness, energy level changes, and different body sensations.

* Emotional level: feelings of anger, fear, sadness, and uneasiness.

* Mental level: overactive or inactive mind.

* Behavioral level: underachieving or overachieving, avoidance, develop-ment of clutter, whining, swearing, unpredictability, and aggressiveness.

* Intuitive level: queer inner feelings and dreams.

The body responds to stress by secreting epinephrine and slowing down digestion. Fats, sugars, and hormones are released in the body, cholesterol rises, blood pressure rises, heartbeat accelerates, muscle tension increas-es, and the blood changes slightly.

Epinephrine production can lead to nutritional deficiencies because it depletes potassium, phosphorus, amino acids, magnesium, and calcium. Under stress, the body doesn't absorb nutrients as well and is unable to replace them correctly. B vitamins and electrolytes, which are essential to the body, are depleted and the growth of free radicals, the cell-destroying agents in the body, is increased.

Stress affects how we look, think and feel. Stress may be classified as physical, emotional, nutritional, and environmental. Physical stress can be caused by many things, including illness, lack of sleep, infections, viruses, bacteria, fungi, and parasites. Emotional stress is caused by negative atti-tudes and emotions such as anger, frustration, worry, grief, and guilt. Nutritional stress can be caused by improper diet or amounts of food, digestive problems, and nutritional deficiencies. Environmental stress can be caused by chemicals, substance abuse, prescription and over-the-counter drugs, and even food preservatives.

For effective stress management:

* Identify the source and level of the stress (physical, emotional, nutritional, environmental, or a combination of sources).

* Acknowledge that the stress is there.

* Take action to control or modify the stress.

* Release the stress.

Since control of all the external circumstances surrounding stress is impossible, it is necessary to handle the circumstances that you can. Changing to a better diet and getting the proper vitamins, minerals, supplements, rest, and exercise can help control stress. On an emotional level learning to balance life between family, work, spirituality, community, intimate relationships, and self with realistic goals and expectations can minimize stress. If an error is made, don't dwell on it or berate yourself, just rectify it as soon as possible. The best defense against stress is a positive attitude. A positive attitude helps all levels of stress. Living in the moment and flowing with life is a better way to control stress than fighting against it.

Relaxation plays a key role in stress reduction. Deep breathing, time off, aromatherapy, hobbies, yoga, tai chi, massage, meditation and self-hypnosis can help keep stress in check.

Stress Relief Remedies

MENTAL ATTITUDE
Cause: fear of change.
Cure: develop positive thought, actions and deeds.

FOODS & DIET
Avoid: alcohol, tobacco, drugs, sugar, caffeine, carbonated drinks, food colorings, additives, preservatives, processed meats and other processed foods; limit dairy foods.
Good Foods: low-fat, high-fiber, mostly vegetarian diet; buttermilk, broccoli, cabbage, cauliflower, tropical fruit, brussels sprouts, apple pectin, kelp, yogurt, artichokes, sardines, grains, oat bran, tuna, swordfish, salmon, turkey, chicken, seeds, nuts, kelp, beans, legumes, squash, spinach, egg yolk, liver, romaine, carob, soybeans.

VITAMINS & SUPPLEMENTS
Multivitamin and mineral supplement with whole foods and enzymes, Vitamin A, E, C, D, B complex, bioflavonoids, calcium, magnesium, potassium, NAC (N-acetylcysteine), L-tyrosine, L-lysine, lecithin, coenzyme Q10, melatonin, selenium, acidophilus.

HERBS
Ginkgo biloba, milk thistle, alfalfa, catnip, hops, coriander, cumin, bilberry, catnip, dong quai, valerian, hops, kava, passionflower, chaparral, red clover, basil, oregano, oat straw.

AROMATHERAPY
Chamomile, frankincense, rose, lavender, eucalyptus, neroli, melissa, sage, benzoin, fennel, peppermint, sandalwood.

The following scripts should be used in the morning and at night for at least six weeks. To optimize results, you may even want to try the scripts for anxiety, or for other appropriate symptoms.

STRESS SCRIPTS

STRESS-BUSTER
Intention: To reduce stress.

Find a comfortable place where you won't be disturbed, and sit in a comfortable chair. Now sit back and relax with both feet on the floor, and place your hands on the armrests of the chair or in your lap — whichever is comfortable for you.

Concentrate as you breathe deeply, letting the air come into your nose and out your mouth. Concentrate and breathe IN with the nose and OUT with the mouth. IN with the nose and OUT with the mouth. And IN with the nose and OUT with the mouth. Now let's concentrate on breathing OUT with the mouth and IN with the nose. And OUT with the mouth and IN with the nose. And OUT with the mouth and IN with the mouth.

(Close your eyes and breathe deeply for two minutes. In these two minutes, think of all the stressful things that are happening to you.

Watch and feel the emotions as they pass. Do not try to stop them. Let the stress and emotions flow without interruption for the full two minutes.)

After two minutes, take a deep breath; feel the peace within you. You have processed all the stress and it is gone. Acknowledge this thought and open your eyes.

THE COUNTRY ROAD
Intention: To eliminate stress.

Find a comfortable place where you won't be disturbed, and sit in a comfortable chair. Now sit back and relax with both feet on the floor, and place your hands on the armrests of the chair or in your lap — whichever is comfortable for you.

Concentrate as you breathe deeply, letting the air come into your nose and out your mouth. Concentrate and breathe IN with the nose and OUT with the mouth. IN with the nose and OUT with the mouth. And IN with the nose and OUT with the mouth. Now let's concentrate on breathing OUT with the mouth and IN with the nose. And OUT with the mouth and IN with the nose. And OUT with the mouth and IN with the mouth.

Imagine you are walking down a country road. Nature is all around you. The birds are singing in the trees. The grass is green and dotted with wildflowers. They smell wonderful as you walk down the road. The sun is shining and the sky is a beautiful blue.

As you walk down the road you sing, and your voice is beautiful and melodic. You are so relaxed and you feel in this moment like you don't have a care in the world.

(Close your eyes for a moment and feel how relaxed you are.)

Look up ahead of you on the road. There are many rocks in front of you blocking your path. There are large and small ones stopping you from being where you want to go. Look at these rocks. On each rock is the name of something that is stopping you from being who you want to be.

You may not be able to read the names but that's okay, you know that these are the things that are stopping you.

(Close your eyes for a moment and look at the rocks.)

You have superhuman strength here. Look to the side of the road; there is a shovel there. Pick up the shovel and start digging a hole. Within a short time you have a hole that is wide enough to fit all of the rocks. Look down the hole; it is a bottomless pit.

(Close your eyes for a moment and look at the pit.)

Go over to the rocks and pick each one up and throw it down into the pit. It doesn't matter how heavy they are — you have superhuman strength and can pick them up easily. Throw the rocks down into the pit one by one by one.

(Close your eyes for a moment and see yourself throw each rock down into the pit.)

When all the rocks are cleared from your path, pick up the shovel and fill in the hole. When the hole is full, stand on top of the hole and jump up and down. You know that your path is clear of any obstacles that were in your way. You take a deep breath and feel all the tension and stress go out of your body, mind, and spirit. You are more relaxed than you have ever known yourself to be.

Feeling happy, start walking down the road. You are so joyful you begin to sing, and you know this feeling will stay with you.

THE MOUNTAIN
Intention: To eliminate stress.

Find a comfortable place where you won't be disturbed, and sit in a comfortable chair. Now sit back and relax with both feet on the floor, and place your hands on the armrests of the chair or in your lap — whichever is comfortable for you.

Concentrate as you breathe deeply, letting the air come into your nose and out your mouth. Concentrate and breathe IN with the nose and OUT with the mouth. IN with the nose and OUT with the mouth. And IN with the nose and OUT with the mouth. Now let's concentrate on breathing OUT with the mouth and IN with the nose. And OUT with the mouth and IN with the nose. And OUT with the mouth and IN with the mouth.

Imagine you are on top of a mountain. The sky around you is dark and filled with dense black clouds. The air is heavy around you. The wind starts to blow. It begins to rain and lightning flashes across the sky.

There is no place to go, and you feel yourself becoming wet as the rain falls down upon you. You feel a deep heaviness all around you.

(Close your eyes for a moment and feel the heaviness.)

Look up at the sky. You see a glimmer of blue sky. It is the most beautiful blue you have ever seen. Keep looking at that patch of blue sky. Watch as that patch of blue sky begins to get bigger and bigger. Now watch as the clouds start rolling away from you.

(Close your eyes for a moment and see the clouds going away.)

You see a ray of sunshine. The sunshine is warm and comforting. Feel the sunshine as the sun breaks through the clouds. Watch as each and every cloud rolls away and the sun comes out, shining brightly. How centered you feel as you begin to relax. So calm as the tension eases out of your body. Everything is so beautiful, clean, and new around you.

(Close your eyes for a moment and feel how relaxed you are.)

Watch as you see rainbows appear all over the sky. Look at all the rainbows and see their bright colors. How beautiful it is as rainbow after rainbow spans the sky. You feel happy and joyful. So positive with all this beauty around you. You know that you are emotionally centered and physically relaxed. Any negative feeling has rolled away with the clouds. Bask in the light of the rainbows, feeling positive, centered and happy. You know this feeling will stay with you.

CHAPTER 38

Tooth Problems

Teeth have an inner part of dentin that is covered by a layer of a very hard substance called enamel. In the center is a pulp cavity and root or roots. The crown (upper part that is above the gum) is covered with hard enamel. The tooth is attached to the jaw by a bonelike substance called cementum. The hard tissues of the tooth function to tear, crush, and grind food. Periodontal tissues (the ones around the teeth) include the bone, cementum, and gingiva (gums), which support the teeth.

Teeth can be affected by various conditions, including dental caries, periodontal disease, and malocclusion. Tooth decay is caused by bacteria and depends on five factors: poor oral hygiene, sugar, poor nutrition, and the vulnerability of the tooth enamel. Plaque — sticky deposits of bacteria, mucus, and food particles — forms a growth medium for bacteria to live in and attack the gums and teeth, unless removed by brushing and flossing.

Periodontal disease is a low-grade, chronic infection that may result in tooth loss because of the recession or loss of the supporting tissues. Gingivitis, or inflammation of the gums, is the beginning of periodontal disease. Badly fitted fillings, too much soft food, and continuous breathing through the mouth can contribute to gingivitis. Gingivitis can also lead to pyorrhea (discharge of pus) or periodontitis (inflammation of tissues around the teeth), which can cause halitosis (bad breath), bleeding or painful gums, and eventually tooth loss.

Abnormal tooth alignment, or malocclusion, means the teeth are positioned badly and don't close properly, which results in chewing difficulty.

Problems in the mouth usually relate to underlying body disorders or nutritional deficiencies. A proper diet, regular dental checkups, brushing with a soft, natural bristle brush, rubbing natural Vitamin E or clove oil on the gums, flossing daily, and changing toothbrushes monthly can help prevent and minimize diseases of the teeth. For toothaches, rinsing the affected area with warm salt water until you can see your dentist may provide some relief. Adequate nutrition during pregnancy and in childhood are important in the development of strong teeth.

Tooth Problem Relief Remedies

MENTAL ATTITUDE

Cause: self-neglect.

Cure: take time for yourself.

FOODS & DIET

Avoid: alcohol, tobacco, drugs, sugar, caffeine, sodas, food colorings, additives, preservatives, processed meats, and other processed foods.

Good Foods: low-fat, high-fiber, mostly vegetarian diet; artichokes, salmon, tuna, kelp, carob, brazil nuts, dandelion greens, soybeans, almonds, spinach, egg yolks, corn oil, flaxseed oil, liver, carrots, coconut, strawberries, brown rice, molasses, rye, cabbage, pineapple, romaine.

VITAMINS & SUPPLEMENTS

Multivitamin and mineral supplement with whole foods and enzymes, Vitamin A, E, C, D, B complex, coenzyme Q10, zinc, selenium, phosphorus, calcium, magnesium, L-lysine, L-cysteine, L-tyrosine, bioflavonoids.

HERBS

Rose hips, clove oil, goldenseal, aloe vera gel, echinacea, cloves, willow, sage.

AROMATHERAPY

Chamomile, camphor, peppermint, sage.

The following scripts should be used in the morning and at night for at least six weeks. To optimize results, you may even want to try the scripts for pain and general illness.

TOOTH PROBLEM SCRIPTS

THE ROSE GARDEN
Intention: To eliminate tooth disease.

Find a comfortable place where you won't be disturbed, and sit in a comfortable chair. Now sit back and relax with both feet on the floor, and place your hands on the armrests of the chair or in your lap — whichever is comfortable for you.

Concentrate as you breathe deeply, letting the air come into your

nose and out your mouth. Concentrate and breathe IN with the nose and OUT with the mouth. IN with the nose and OUT with the mouth. And IN with the nose and OUT with the mouth. Now let's concentrate on breathing OUT with the mouth and IN with the nose. And OUT with the mouth and IN with the nose. And OUT with the mouth and IN with the mouth.

Imagine you are in a rose garden. Everything is so serene and quiet. The garden is manicured and neat and you know that this is a very special place. Look at the roses. There are so many different colors. Breathe in the fragrance. It is so nice and relaxing. As you breathe in the aroma of the roses, you start to become centered, calm, and very, very relaxed.

(Close your eyes for a moment and feel how relaxed you are.)

Go over to one of the roses and look at it. It is very beautiful. Look closer at the rose and you see very tiny bugs eating into the rose's petals. The more you look at the rose, the more bugs you see.

Look over to your right. There is a spray bottle of liquid there. Pick it up and spray the rose petals that have the bugs on them. Watch as the bugs disappear. Watch as the spray from the bottle gets rid of each bug, one by one.

(Close your eyes for a moment and see the bugs disappearing.)

As this rose becomes bug-free, look at the other roses on this bush. Wherever you find any bugs on the roses, use your spray bottle to make them disappear. Do this until every bug is gone from every rose.

(Close your eyes for a moment and see the bugs disappearing.)

Now look at the leaves and roots of this rosebush. There are a lot of bugs there. They have chewed near the roots of the rosebush. There are holes in the leaves. Use your spray bottle to make these bugs disappear. Watch as each bug disappears when the spray hits it. Continue to spray until the entire rosebush is free from the bugs.

(Close your eyes for a moment and see the bugs disappearing.)

Now look at all the holes the bugs have left in the rose petals, the leaves, and near the roots of the bush. Look to your left; there is a magic wand there. Pick up the wand and point it. A ray of golden healing light is emitted from the wand's tip. You know you can use this magic wand to make the rosebush whole and healthy again. You can repair all the holes in the petals and leaves. You can heal the roots and all the damage to the whole bush. Point the magic wand at the rosebush. Watch the golden light come out of the wand. See the healing taking place. Do this until the rosebush is healthy and strong again, perfect in every way.

(Close your eyes for a moment and see the healing taking place.)

Look at how perfect the rosebush is now. You are happy and content. There is a bench in the garden. Taking the spray bottle and magic wand with you, walk over to the bench and sit down. You become very relaxed and comfortable. You know you are going to use the spray bottle with the healing liquid and magic wand to heal your teeth. Everything is safe and nontoxic to you. Point the spray bottle into your mouth and spray. Feel the magic liquid help to heal your disease. Feel how any problems are being healed. The cause of your problem is just disappearing in this healing spray. Turn the magic wand and point it towards your mouth. Feel the healing light repairing, fixing, mending any damage. Making your teeth, your gums, your roots strong and perfect.

Your mouth, teeth, and gums are becoming healthy, strong and whole. Continue to use the magic spray and magic wand as long as you need to. Feel the problems disappearing. Feel the healing taking place.

(Close your eyes for a moment and heal your teeth, gums, and mouth.)

Feel how your mouth, your teeth, and your gums are whole and healthy. Feel how strong your teeth are. Your gums are pink and healthy. You are happy and thankful for the healing that has taken place. You know that your teeth, gums, and mouth have healed. This feeling will stay with you.

THE TOOTH
Intention: To eliminate tooth pain.

Find a comfortable place where you won't be disturbed, and sit in a comfortable chair. Now sit back and relax with both feet on the floor, and place your hands on the armrests of the chair or in your lap — whichever is comfortable for you.

Concentrate as you breathe deeply, letting the air come into your nose and out your mouth. Concentrate and breathe IN with the nose and OUT with the mouth. IN with the nose and OUT with the mouth.

And IN with the nose and OUT with the mouth. Now let's concentrate on breathing OUT with the mouth and IN with the nose. And OUT with the mouth and IN with the nose. And OUT with the mouth and IN with the mouth.

Imagine that you are very, very tiny and that you are inside your tooth. You feel very safe, and the tooth that you are inside of is very white and pretty. Look around at the inside of your tooth. Look for the source of your pain. As you find it, notice that the color is different. Walk over to the spot where the pain is and look at the color. See how different it is.

(Close your eyes for a moment and see the source of your pain.)

Reach in your pocket. You find a golden paintbrush there. It is a magic paintbrush that can change the color of the painful spot to white. It can heal the pain spot and take away any pain. As you look at the golden paintbrush, you know it will automatically dispense the right amount of paint that you need. There is an endless supply of paint in this paintbrush and you can never run out. Take the paintbrush and start painting the place that is a different color. You are painting away the source of your pain. See how the spot immediately turns white as you use your paintbrush. You feel any pain just disappear. Continue painting as long as you need to. You know that each brushstroke is taking away the pain.

(Close your eyes for a moment and paint away your pain.)

Now go to any other spots in any of your teeth that need healing and paint the pain away. Each tooth feels healthy and whole. They feel strong and white. You know the healing is taking place.

When you are done, place the golden paintbrush back inside your pocket. You feel positive, happy and pain-free. You know this feeling will stay with you.

CHAPTER 39

Ulcers

Stress ulcers are acute lesions caused by trauma, burns, major surgery, and central nervous system disease. They occur in the stomach or duodenum as multiple, shallow bleeding erosions. Peptic ulcers are the pitting or ulceration of the mucous membrane of the esophagus, stomach, or duodenum (the first part of the small intestine that proceeds from the stomach). Possible causes of peptic ulcers are the infectious bacteria *Helicobacter pylori*, anxiety, aspirin, anti-inflammatory drugs, steroids, stress, and food allergies. The symptoms of ulcer may include a chronic gnawing, burning pain which occurs after eating, lower back pain, headaches, nausea, and itching.

Gastric juices consist of hydrochloric acid, mucus, and pepsin. If the gastric juices act on the wall of the digestive tract, a peptic ulcer will occur. When the stomach lining doesn't protect itself from the acidic gastric juices, the acids start to digest the stomach itself.

Proper diet – including avoidance of alcohol, fried foods, strong spices, carbonated drinks, and dairy products; eating soft foods; and drinking purified water – can help.

Traditional treatment includes antibiotics and drug therapy that blocks the acids. Don't forget to research the side effects. Certain types of prescription and over-the-counter drugs disrupt the normal digestion process, which may create malabsorption of food. These drugs may also alter the function of the stomach lining, and provide only temporary relief that masks the problem. Natural remedies include a proper diet, aromatherapy, acupuncture, homeopathy, herbal therapy, relaxation methods, visualization, and self-hypnosis.

Ulcer Relief Remedies
MENTAL ATTITUDE
Cause: worry or anxiety.
Cure: live in the moment.
FOODS & DIET
Avoid: alcohol, tobacco, nicotine, aspirin, caffeine, carbonated drinks, salt, animal fats, cow's milk, spicy foods, raw fruit, food colorings, additives, preservatives, white flour, white rice, turnips, radishes, brussels

sprouts, broccoli, cauliflower, processed meats, processed foods.
Good Foods: low-fat, high-fiber, mostly vegetarian diet; cabbage juice, bananas, pectin, brown rice, whole grains, vegetables, avocados, yams, potatoes, squash, yogurt.

VITAMINS & SUPPLEMENTS
Multivitamin and mineral supplement with whole foods and enzymes, Vitamin A, E, K, B complex, zinc, bromelain, acidophilus, L-glutamine, essential fatty acids.

HERBS
Aloe vera juice, meadowsweet, licorice root, slippery elm, ginger, alfalfa, cat's claw, marshmallow root, hops, sage.

AROMATHERAPY
Lavender, myrrh, geranium, eucalyptus, chamomile.

The following scripts should be used in the morning and at night for at least six weeks. To optimize results, you may even want to try the scripts for anxiety, stress, pain, and general illness.

ULCER SCRIPTS

THE METAL EGG
Intention: To eliminate ulcers.

Find a comfortable place where you won't be disturbed, and sit in a comfortable chair. Now sit back and relax with both feet on the floor, and place your hands on the armrests of the chair or in your lap — whichever is comfortable for you.

Concentrate as you breathe deeply, letting the air come into your nose and out your mouth. Concentrate and breathe IN with the nose and OUT with the mouth. IN with the nose and OUT with the mouth. And IN with the nose and OUT with the mouth. Now let's concentrate on breathing OUT with the mouth and IN with the nose. And OUT with the mouth and IN with the nose. And OUT with the mouth and IN with the mouth.

Imagine you are inside a hollow metal egg. You are standing in the middle and have a flashlight with you. Shine your flashlight over the inside surface of the egg. The surface is gold. Everywhere around you the glossy surface shimmers and shines in your light. All the areas are as smooth as glass. Look to your right; on the floor you see some small holes.

(Close your eyes for a moment and see these holes.)

Shine your flashlight on these holes. You see a liquid in the center of each hole. The liquid is bubbling and steaming. Watch as the liquid bubbles and steams in each hole. As you look, you see each hole become larger. The liquid in each hole seems to be eating away the sides of each hole, making it bigger.

(Close your eyes for a moment and see the holes getting larger.)

Look down to your left; there is a small bottle with a cap on it. You somehow know that placing a couple of drops of liquid from this bottle into each hole will neutralize the bubbling acid. Pick up the bottle and take off the cap. Go over to each hole and place a couple of drops of the bottle's liquid into one of the holes. Watch as the bubbling in each hole stops. Watch and feel how the liquid in the hole seems to be drying up and finally disappears. Now watch as the hole repairs itself. See the hole disappear and how the shiny gold metal of the surface is unbroken. Watch the hole disappear, leaving a shiny, glossy surface. Go over to each hole and heal each one.

(Close your eyes for a moment and see and feel the healing taking place.)

When you are done, shine your flashlight all around the metal egg. Look at its sides, the ceiling. Wherever you find a hole, repair it with the liquid. Do this until the whole inside of the metal egg is repaired.

Run your hands over the surface of the metal egg. Feel how smooth and unbroken it is. You have repaired this egg and you feel happy, health, and pain-free. You know these feelings will stay with you.

THE ROOMS
Intention: To eliminate ulcers.

Find a comfortable place where you won't be disturbed, and sit in a comfortable chair. Now sit back and relax with both feet on the floor, and place your hands on the armrests of the chair or in your lap — whichever is comfortable for you.

Concentrate as you breathe deeply, letting the air come into your nose and out your mouth. Concentrate and breathe IN with the nose and OUT with the mouth. IN with the nose and OUT with the mouth.

And IN with the nose and OUT with the mouth. Now let's concentrate on breathing OUT with the mouth and IN with the nose. And OUT with the mouth and IN with the nose. And OUT with the mouth and IN with the mouth.

Imagine that you are watching a magic TV. The room is well-lit and you are sitting in a very comfortable chair. On the screen is a picture of your stomach. You can see where your ulcers are on the screen. As you watch the screen, you see a white light come into your stomach. Watch how this light begins to kill the bacteria and balance all your gastric acids. The white light is balancing all the acids to be exactly right for you.

(Close your eyes for a moment and see the white light balancing.)

Now watch as the white light soothes your cells and any other problems that are physically creating the ulcers.

Feel the healing taking place. Feel the balancing and repair of all your digestive tract. Watch and feel how healthy this area is. Now watch as the white light repairs your stomach lining. Making your stomach lining whole and perfect, right now.

(Close your eyes for a moment and see and feel the healing.)

Look at the screen and see that your stomach is in proper working order. You feel, trust, and know this.

Get up off the chair and walk into the next room. In front of you there is a table. The table contains all the right foods to keep your stomach healthy. Look at these foods, and as you do you feel a desire for these foods. These are the foods that you want and need. These healthy foods are the ones you crave. These foods that will keep your body in perfect working order. You desire only the right amounts of these wonderful, healthy foods. You know that these foods will keep you healthy.

(Close your eyes for a moment and see all the healthy foods.)

Walk out of this room and go to the room at your left. There is a jacuzzi there. The water is bubbling and the temperature is exactly right for you. The aroma from the jacuzzi is so relaxing and soothing. Take off your clothes and go into the jacuzzi. Feel the swirling, bubbling water take away all your stress, all your tension. You are becoming more and more relaxed. Feel how every part of your body and mind just quiets down and relaxes.

(Close your eyes for a moment and feel the relaxation.)

Now feel how healthy and relaxed you are. Feel the energy come into your body. Making your body strong, your mind clear, your spirit happy. You feel so good. You know this feeling will stay with you.

CHAPTER 40

Vertigo and Dizziness

Vertigo is a sensation of dizziness, lightheadedness, a feeling as if the person is spinning, or a sensation of an imminent loss of consciousness. There is an impaired sense of equilibrium or balance. A sense of balance relies on a combination of visual input from the eyes and mechanisms in the inner ear. Dizziness may not always be a symptom of vertigo.

When the central nervous system receives different messages from the eye, muscle, skin, and inner ear receptors, vertigo can occur. It can also result from hyperventilation, substance abuse, motion sickness, anxiety or stress, fear of heights, anemia, viral infections, nutritional deficiencies, too much sodium, high or low blood pressure, brain tumors, head injury, poor circulation, and fever.

Aging may affect vertigo. Bits of debris can accumulate in the inner ears, which could have an impact on sending false signals to the brain. Also nerve impulses to the brain slow down with the aging process and this could cause loss of balance or dizziness upon sudden movement.

To stop dizziness, sit in a chair, place both feet on the floor, and stare at a fixed object for a few minutes. Hand and eye coordination exercises like throwing and catching a ball can improve your reflexes for a quicker recovery time when dizziness occurs.

Natural remedies include a proper diet, aromatherapy, acupuncture, homeopathy, herbal, vitamin, and supplement therapy, relaxation methods, visualization, and self-hypnosis.

Vertigo and Dizziness Relief Remedies

MENTAL ATTITUDE
Cause: refusal to face conditions around self.
Cure: stop fear, use positive thought, and take action.

FOODS & DIET
Avoid: alcohol, nicotine, caffeine, salt, food colorings, additives, preservatives, fried foods, processed meats, other processed foods.
Good Foods: low-fat, high-fiber, mostly vegetarian diet.

VITAMINS & SUPPLEMENTS

Multivitamin and mineral supplement with whole foods and enzymes, manganese, Vitamin A, C, E, bioflavonoids, calcium, lecithin, magnesium, B complex, iron, chromium picolinate, choline, inositol, coenzyme Q10, zinc, melatonin, kelp.

HERBS

Ginger, ginkgo biloba, ginseng, cayenne, butcher's broom, dandelion.

AROMATHERAPY

Basil, black pepper, lavender, melissa, peppermint, rosemary.

The following scripts should be used in the morning and at night for at least six weeks. To optimize results, you may even want to try the scripts for anxiety, stress, and general illness.

VERTIGO AND DIZZINESS SCRIPTS

THE MAGIC LEAF
Intention: To eliminate vertigo and dizziness.

Find a comfortable place where you won't be disturbed, and sit in a comfortable chair. Now sit back and relax with both feet on the floor, and place your hands on the armrests of the chair or in your lap — whichever is comfortable for you.

Concentrate as you breathe deeply, letting the air come into your nose and out your mouth. Concentrate and breathe IN with the nose and OUT with the mouth. IN with the nose and OUT with the mouth. And IN with the nose and OUT with the mouth. Now let's concentrate on breathing OUT with the mouth and IN with the nose. And OUT with the mouth and IN with the nose. And OUT with the mouth and IN with the mouth.

Imagine you are in a boat on a very calm lake. Look towards the horizon; it looks so beautiful. The water of the lake is calm and still. It is clear and you can see to the bottom. The sky is blue with some fluffy white clouds. How wonderful to just drift in this boat without a care or worry in the world.

There is a small current in the lake that moves your boat. Look into this current and see a small leaf drifting along with you. Reach down into the water and pick up this leaf. You are so relaxed and calm.

(Close your eyes for a moment and feel how relaxed you are.)

Now feel the current getting faster, and as it does your boat begins to go faster. Look in front of you. There is a whirlpool there. You are holding onto the leaf. It is a magic leaf and the colors are so beautiful. Watch and feel the boat enter into the whirlpool. Feel the boat start spinning. As the boat starts to spin faster in the whirlpool, you realize that you are not spinning. Look at the leaf. You feel centered and calm. Even though the boat is spinning, you are not. You know that the magic leaf is making you steady, strong. Nothing around you is moving, even though the boat is moving beneath you. You trust and feel this.

(Close your eyes for a moment and feel how steady you are.)

Look down at the boat and see it spinning beneath you. Look up and you realize that you are not spinning. Look closer and see how calm and centered you are. Holding on to this magic leaf makes you unaffected by the spinning that is all around you. You feel wonderful. You know that anytime you need this magic leaf it will appear in your hand. It will make you calm, centered, steady, strong. The leaf will make any dizziness subside, at any time.

You feel and know this and are very happy. You know that this steady, balanced feeling will stay with you.

FIREWORKS
Intention: To eliminate vertigo and dizziness.

Find a comfortable place where you won't be disturbed, and sit in a comfortable chair. Now sit back and relax with both feet on the floor, and place your hands on the armrests of the chair or in your lap — whichever is comfortable for you.

Concentrate as you breathe deeply, letting the air come into your nose and out your mouth. Concentrate and breathe IN with the nose and OUT with the mouth. IN with the nose and OUT with the mouth. And IN with the nose and OUT with the mouth. Now let's concentrate on breathing OUT with the mouth and IN with the nose. And

OUT with the mouth and IN with the nose. And OUT with the mouth and IN with the mouth.

Imagine you are standing in the center of a golden room. The ceiling, the walls, the floor are all gold. There is nothing in this room. Look to your left and see a door.

Sit down on the floor in the middle of the room. Watch the walls and ceiling. Fireworks in beautiful colors start to emerge. You are centered and calm and know this is a safe place. Watch the spectacular display of colors as they burst all around you. It is so very beautiful.

(Close your eyes for a moment and look at the fireworks.)

Watch as the fireworks all turn to emerald green. You know this is a healing color. Feel the light of the emerald green fireworks enter into your body. Feel your body balance. Feel your body becoming centered, making you calm. Feel how your nerves are becoming balanced. Everything is healing. Watch and feel how the light goes into your eyes, your ears, your brain. You know this green light is balancing you, centering you, healing you. Healing anything that is wrong with your body right now.

(Close your eyes for a moment and feel the healing.)

Now watch as the fireworks become many colors again. The colors are becoming so intense. Feel the air become heavy around you. Look down at your body. You have emerald green light all around you. It is surrounding every part of your body. It is keeping you calm, centered, relaxed, and in balance.

(Close your eyes for a moment and feel how balanced you are.)

Get up off the floor and go to the door in the room. Look down at your body and see the healing green light. You know this light will stay with you, keeping you calm, relaxed, centered, and balanced.

HERB AND PLANT COMMON AND LATIN NAMES

alfalfa (*Medicago sativa*)

aloe vera (*Aloe vera*). Avoid during pregnancy; avoid all high doses.

angelica (*Angelica archangelica*). Avoid large doses during pregnancy.

arnica (*Arnica montana*). Do not use on broken skin; best used topically.

astragalus (*Astragalus membranaceus*).

basil (*Ocimum basilicum*). Avoid during pregnancy.

bearberry. *See* **uva ursi**

bilberry (*Vaccinium myrtillus*). Avoid if diabetic.

black cohosh (*Cimicifuga racemosa*).

blue cohosh (*Caulophylum thaictroides*). Avoid during first and second trimesters of pregnancy.

boneset (*Eupatorium perfoliatum*). Avoid high doses.

buchu (*Agathosma betulina, A. crenulata*)

burdock root (*Articum lappa*)

butcher's broom (*Ruscus aculeatus*).

cabbage (*Brassica oleracea*).

California poppy (*Eschscholzia californica*)

catnip (*Nepeta catarina*)

cat's claw or **uña del gato** (*Uncaria tomentosa*).

cayenne pepper (*Capsicum frutescens*). Avoid during pregnancy and breastfeeding.

chamomile (*Matricaria chamomilla*). Avoid during pregnancy.

chaparral (*Larrea tridentata*). Avoid high doses.

chaste berry. *See* **vitex**

chaste tree. *See* **vitex**.

cilantro. *See* **coriander**.

cinnamon (*Cinnamomum* spp.). Avoid during pregnancy.

coriander (Chinese parsley, cilantro) (*Coriandrum sativum*).

cowslip (*Primula veris*). Avoid high doses during pregnancy.

cranberry (*Vaccinium macrocarpon*).

cumin (*Cuminum cyminum*).

damiana (*Turnera diffusa*).

dandelion (*Taraxacum officinale*).

dill (*Anethum graveolens*).

dong quai (*Angelica sinensis*)

echinacea (purple coneflower) (*Echinacea* spp.)

Essiac tea (several herbs, usually burdock root, sheep sorrel, turkey rhubarb root, slippery elm bark).

false unicorn (*Chamaelirium luteum*).

fennel (*Foeniculum volgare*). Avoid high doses during pregnancy.

fenugreek (*Trigonella foenum-graceum*). Avoid if diabetic or pregnant.

feverfew (*Tanacetum parthenium*). Avoid with hypertension, pregnancy, or if taking blood-thinning drugs.

figwort (*Scrophularia nodosa*). Avoid if rapid heartbeat is present.

garcinia cambogia (*Garcinia cambogia*).

garlic (*Allium sativum*).

ginger (*Zingiber officinalis*). Use low doses during pregnancy.

ginkgo (gingko) (*Ginkgo biloba*). Avoid high dosages.

ginseng (*Panax ginseng*). Avoid high dosages and prolonged use if you are pregnant or have hypertension.

goldenseal (*Hydrastis canadensis*). Avoid during pregnancy or hypertension.

gotu kola (*Centella asiatica*).

hawthorn (hawthorn berries) (*Cratageus* spp.)

heartsease (*Viola* spp.). Avoid high doses.

hops (*Humulus lupulus*). Avoid if in depression.

horehound (*Marrubium vulgare*).

horsetail (*Equisetum* spp.). Avoid during heavy menstrual bleeding.

hyssop (*Hyssopus officinalis*). Avoid high doses.

juniper (*Juniperus communis*). Avoid long-term use and during pregnancy.

kava (*Piper methysticum*).

lady's mantle (*Alchemilla xanthochlora, A. vulgaris*). Avoid during pregnancy.

lavender (*Lavandula angustifolia*). Avoid high doses during pregnancy

lemon balm (*Melissa officinalis*).

licorice root (*Glycorrhiza* spp.) Avoid high doses during pregnancy.

lobelia (*Lobelia inflata*). Avoid with hypertension and avoid large doses.

marjoram (*Origanum majorana*).

marshmallow (*Althaea officinalis*).

meadowsweet (*Filipendula ulmaria*).

milk thistle (*Silybum marianum*).

mint (*Mentha* spp.).

motherwort (*Leonurus cardiaca*). Avoid if pregnant or if you have a heart condition.

mugwort (*Artemisia vulgaris*). Avoid during pregnancy and breastfeeding.

myrrh (*Commiphora molmol*). Avoid during pregnancy.

nettle (stinging nettle) (*Urtica dioica*).
nutmeg (*Myristica fragrans*). Avoid high doses.

passion flower (*Passiflora incarnata*).
pau d'arco (*Tabebuia heptaphylla*).

raspberry leaf (*Rubus idaeus*).
red clover (*Trifolium pratense*).
rosemary (*Rosmarinus officinalis*).

sage (*Salvia officinalis*). Avoid high doses during pregnancy
or if epileptic.
saw palmetto (*Serenoa repens*).
sheep sorrel (*Rumex acetosella*).
skullcap (*Scutellaria laterifolia* and species).
slippery elm (*Ulmus rubra*).
St. John's wort (*Hypericum perforatum*).

tea tree (*Melaleuca alternifolia*).
thyme (*Thymus vulgaris*). Avoid high doses during pregnancy.
turkey rhubarb (*Rheum palmatum*).
turmeric (*Curcuma longa*)

uva ursi (bearberry) (*Arctostaphylos uva-ursi*).
valerian (*Valeriana officinalis* and species). Avoid with sleeping
medications, and do not take for more than 2 to 3 weeks.
vervain (*Verbena officinalis*). Avoid during pregnancy. Can be
taken during labor.
vitex (chaste berry, chaste tree) (*Vitex agnus-castus*). Avoid
during pregnancy.

wild lettuce (*Latuca virosa*).
wild oats (*Avena sativa*).

wild yam *(Dioscorea villosa)* Avoid during pregnancy.

willow bark (white willow) *(Salix alba)*.

wood betony *(Stachys betonica)*. Avoid during pregnancy.

yarrow *(Achillea millefolium)*. Avoid large doses during pregnancy.

yellow dock *(Rumex crispus)*.

yucca *(Yucca* spp.).

Index